RN's
Study Guide
NURSING ESSENTIALS

Vicky Li, RN, BA

WITHDRAWN

JONES & BARTLETT
LEARNING

World Headquarters
Jones & Bartlett Learning
5 Wall Street
Burlington, MA 01803
978-443-5000
info@jblearning.com
www.jblearning.com

Jones & Bartlett Learning books and products are available through most bookstores and online booksellers. To contact Jones & Bartlett Learning directly, call 800-832-0034, fax 978-443-8000, or visit our website, www.jblearning.com.

Substantial discounts on bulk quantities of Jones & Bartlett Learning publications are available to corporations, professional associations, and other qualified organizations. For details and specific discount information, contact the special sales department at Jones & Bartlett Learning via the above contact information or send an email to specialsales@jblearning.com.

Production Credits

VP, Executive Publisher: David D. Cella
Executive Editor: Amanda Martin
Acquisitions Editor: Teresa Reilly
Editorial Assistant: Emma Huggard
Production Editor: Vanessa Richards
Marketing Communications Manager: Katie Hennessy
Product Fulfillment Manager: Wendy Kilborn
Composition: S4Carlisle Publishing Services
Cover Design: Kristin E. Parker
Rights & Media Specialist: Wes DeShano
Cover Image: Top: © elic/Shutterstock; Bottom: © Daniel Lohmer/Shutterstock
Printing and Binding: Edwards Brothers Malloy
Cover Printing: Edwards Brothers Malloy

Library of Congress Cataloging-in-Publication Data

Names: Li, Vicky, author.
Title: RN's study guide: nursing essentials / Vicky Li.
Description: First edition. | Burlington, MA: Jones & Bartlett Learning, [2018] | Includes bibliographical references and index.
Identifiers: LCCN 2016031311 | ISBN 9781284115970 (pbk.)
Subjects: | MESH: Nursing Care | Signs and Symptoms
Classification: LCC RT41 | NLM WY 100.1 | DDC 610.73--dc23 LC record available at https://lccn.loc.gov/2016031311

6048

Printed in the United States of America
20 19 18 17 16   10 9 8 7 6 5 4 3 2 1

Contents

CONTENTS

CONTENTS

CONTENTS

CONTENTS

Disclaimer

There may be images in this book that feature models; these models do not necessarily endorse, represent, or participate in the activities represented in the images. Any screenshots in this product are for educational and instructive purposes only. Any individuals and scenarios featured in the case studies throughout this product may be real or fictitious, but are used for instructional purposes only.

The authors, editor, and publisher have made every effort to provide accurate information. However, they are not responsible for errors, omissions, or for any outcomes related to the use of the contents of this book and take no responsibility for the use of the products and procedures described. Treatments and side effects described in this book may not be applicable to all people; likewise, some people may require a dose or experience a side effect that is not described herein. Drugs and medical devices are discussed that may have limited availability controlled by the Food and Drug Administration (FDA) for use only in a research study or clinical trial. Research, clinical practice, and government regulations often change the accepted standard in this field. When consideration is being given to use of any drug in the clinical setting, the health care provider or reader is responsible for determining FDA status of the drug, reading the package insert, and reviewing prescribing information for the most up-to-date recommendations on dose, precautions, and contraindications, and determining the appropriate usage for the product. This is especially important in the case of drugs that are new or seldom used.

Preface

RN's Study Guide: Nursing Essentials aims to present nursing fundamentals in the simplest way possible to facilitate in-depth study. It is designed to help time-pressed students get the gist of an otherwise overwhelming amount of abstruse information, and to aid them in passing academic tests and realizing their career goals.

From a nurse's perspective, this text stresses nursing priorities. It offers highlighted tips, along with succinct rationales. The user-friendly format makes it easy to retain the important knowledge needed to provide optimal care for patients and families.

Any readers interested in healthcare basics should also find this book informative. Note, however, that reproductive, pediatric, and mental health issues are beyond the scope of this book. Moreover, it does not include reference values or complicated aspects of experts' care decisions, such as classifications, diagnostic processes, and medical interventions.

The content is organized by body system. Each chapter starts with "Anatomic Pointers," proceeds to alphabetically listed "Disorders and Conditions," and, where needed, provides an additional section, "Other Pointers and Concerns." Each section on a disorder or condition comprises up to five subsections: a brief introduction to the disorder/condition, "Main Symptoms," "Selected Nursing Tips," "Points to Consider," and "Precautions."

This book is not intended to be a clinical guide. In a broad sense, however, any nursing material is clinically based, and nursing principles may be applicable in different scenarios under similar circumstances. Thus, the nurse needs to know why, not just how.

Medical conditions can be extremely complicated. Many disorders affect and are affected by multiple systems, with causes and features overlapping or intermingling. In addition, the unique particulars of each patient's circumstance must be taken into consideration before a prudent decision can be made—whether on a test or in a clinical setting. Referring to the most recent data is imperative, as the science continues to advance with each passing day.

Readers will be better prepared to meet the challenges they are likely to face, academically at school or professionally at work, when they are equipped with these nursing essentials to deepen their understanding of nursing dynamics.

Acknowledgments

RN's Study Guide: Nursing Essentials was inspired by the more than a dozen source books listed in the Selected Bibliography. First, I want to give credit to all these authors; any omissions are unintentional.

Embarking on a project that involved condensing an enormous amount of material into a brief volume was definitely an audacious decision. I would be lying if I said the scope or the topics of the book did not intimidate or frustrate me from time to time. In fact, I put this work aside for a whole year and instead wrote a collection of six books of verse (mostly for children). Without the encouragement and support of many professionals, I would have quit many times over. I am deeply grateful to my kind supporters, expert reviewers, and insightful/dedicated editors for making this work possible.

I owe an immense debt of gratitude to Dr. Peter T. Walling, a retired anesthesiologist who is still lecturing all over the world, for his willingness to review chapters and contribute his expertise.

I am extremely grateful to Dr. Elizabeth Seymour, a family doctor and telemedicine physician, who owns two busy clinics, for reviewing several chapters and for her input and support.

My heartfelt thanks to Dr. Russell W. Snook, an ophthalmologist, for his review of and contributions to the eye section, and to Dr. Thomas Cadenhead, an otolaryngologist, for reviewing the ear-related text. Special thanks to Dr. Ron Hellstern, a medical practice management consultant and retired emergency physician, for his invaluable advice.

These doctors managed to find the time in their tight schedules to contribute their expertise to this book. Their time and assistance have meant the world to me. It is their recognition that gave me the strength to finish this often-challenging project.

Having taught for 16 years (in both China and Texas) before becoming a registered nurse, I particularly admire my former nursing instructors. The lessons they taught me, including "warnings" in both my licensed vocational nurse (LVN) and registered nurse (RN) programs, have stayed with me during my 20 years' nursing practice. My sincere thanks to Dr. Sharon L. Van Sell, EdD, RN, PAHM, for her attention, reviewing, and insight.

I greatly appreciate the support I have received from many other professionals as well. Among them are Marty Richardson, MSN, RN, a nursing instructor and a contributor to this book; Daphne Salazar, RN, BSN, CRRN, a hospital nurse; Maria Lourdes Kunkel, MSN, CNOR, an army nurse; Annette Maillard, a nursing educator; Mary Kuhfeldt, a dietician; and Jennifer Patrick and Kathy Yoder, dialysis nurses. They graciously reviewed many chapters or sections. Thanks also to Barbara Blanks, a poet, for her suggestion of separating eye disorders from ear problems in the sensory issues chapter.

My sincere thanks also go to the members of my local writers' critique group: Robert Koger, Helen Schenk, Jacqueline Stem, B. C. Groves, Bill Kincaid, and Don Oldham. Their great patience and helpful suggestions kept me going until its completion. B. C. even said, "I wish I had this book 40 years ago. I want this book. You've sold one!" Her comment was an enormous energy booster for me.

I would also acknowledge the help of my son, Jim Lee, an RN. His reminders and tools—the lab and drug reference books—often came in handy.

I want to give my deepest thanks to Betsy (Elizabeth) Pinter Lowe, a senior editor at a major medical publishing company

(Wolters Kluwer), for an approving nod at the content of a sample chapter and her referral.

I owe special thanks to acquisitions editors Shannon Magee (at Wolters Kluwer), Amanda Martin, Teresa Reilly, and project editor Vanessa Richards for having faith in this project and giving me many pointers, including relaying the positive and constructive feedback of reviewers across the country.

I certainly have a great admiration for my copyeditor, Jill Hobbs, the cover designer, Kristin Parker, and the rights and media specialist, Wesley DeShano. I do appreciate their hard work! Many thanks are due to Danielle Bessette, Lauren Vaughn, and Escaline Aarthi for being my source of support and assistance.

To all the experts and professionals who provide me with valuable resources and helped me in this bold endeavor, I am truly indebted!

—*Vicky Li*

Contributors

Marty Richardson, MSN, RN
Grayson County College
Sherman, Texas

Elizabeth Seymour, MD
Medical Associates
    of Denton, Texas

Russell William Snook, MD
Lewisville, TX

Peter T. Walling, BSc, MB,
    BS (United Kingdom),
    MD (United States),
    FRCA (United Kingdom)
Bartonville, Texas

Advisor

Ron A. Hellstern, MD, FACEP
Irving, Texas

Reviewers

Janet J. Adams, MSN, RT
    (ARRT), RN-ONC
Instructor
Southeast Missouri State
    University
Cape Girardeau, Missouri

Gloria Browning, PhD, RN
Nursing Professor
University of Tennessee,
    Martin
Martin, Tennessee

Rachel W. Cozort, PhD, MSN,
    RN, CNE
Assistant Professor
    of Nursing
Pfeiffer University
Misenheimer, North Carolina

Kimberly Dudas, PhD, RN,
    ANP-BC, CNE
Associate Dean
New Jersey City University
Jersey City, New Jersey

Aida L. Egues, DNP,
    RN-APHN-BC, CNE
Associate Professor of
    Nursing
New York City College of
    Technology of the City
    University of New York
Brooklyn, New York

Shar Georgesen, PhDc, MSN, RN
Associate Professor
Nylen School of Nursing
Morningside College
Sioux City, Iowa

Margaret (Peg) Gramas,
   EdD, MSN, RN
Instructor
Morton College
Cicero, Illinois

Vicki E. Long, DNP, RN, CNM
Assistant Professor
University of South
   Carolina, Aiken
Aiken, South Carolina

Emily A. Newman, MSN, MEd,
   RN, CPE
Simulation/Skills Lab
   Coordinator
Instructor in Nursing
Robert E. Smith School
   of Nursing
Delta State University
Cleveland, Mississippi

LaDonna Northington, LN, DNS
Program Director
Medical Center School of Nursing
University of Mississippi
Jackson, Mississippi

Paul Pope, CNE, MSN, RN
Professor, Nursing Instructor
Mercy College of Nursing
Southwest Baptist University
Springfield, Missouri

Deborah S. Rushing, DNP, RN
Assistant Professor
School of Nursing
Troy University
Troy, Alabama

Nancy Steffen, RN, MSN, CNE
Nursing Instructor
Century College
White Bear Lake, Minnesota

Sharon L. Van Sell, EdD,
   RN, PAHM
Professor
T. Boone Pickens Institute
   of Health Sciences, Dallas
   Center
The Houston J. and Florence A.
   Doswell College of Nursing
Texas Woman's University
Dallas, Texas

Theresa L. Wenzig, RN, MSN
Nursing Faculty
Chemeketa Community College
Salem, Oregon

Polly Gerber Zimmermann,
   RN, MS, MBA, CEN, FAEN
Associate Professor
City College of Chicago
Chicago, Illinois

Foreword

RN's Study Guide: Nursing Essentials is, by its very nature, a condensed and fact-filled narrative.

As a medical student, I transcribed shorthand notes into a pocket-sized desk diary, then memorized them on the underground train traveling to London every day. I found this method of revision extremely effective. Fifty years later, I still own the notebook. In this book, Vicky Li has done all the hard work for you.

Remember that this is a study guide, however—not a medical textbook. It is not suggested that you pick it up and try to read straight through it the day before your exams.

I wish you well with your careers. I have worked with nurses for 50 years in the operating room and know full well how valuable they are to the successful outcomes of medical treatment.

Peter T. Walling, BSc, MB, BS, MD, FRCA
Bartonville, Texas

CHAPTER 1

Hematologic and Immunologic Issues

ANATOMIC POINTERS

In the hematologic system, blood performs a variety of essential functions. It continuously transports oxygen, nutrients, hormones, antibodies, and other substances around the body for use. It also carries cellular-metabolism wastes to sites where they are transformed or eliminated from the body. While circulating through the vascular system, blood helps regulate fluid, electrolyte, and acid-base balance. It can also protect the body with its clotting capability and by fighting infections.

The two major components of the blood are plasma and blood cells. Plasma is the liquid portion of the blood. It consists primarily of water, but also includes proteins (e.g., albumin, globulin), clotting factors (e.g., fibrinogen), electrolytes, nutrients, wastes, and other substances. Within the vascular system, the protein albumin plays an important role in maintaining fluid balance. The presence of sufficient albumin in the plasma creates an osmotic force (colloidal or oncotic pressure) that offsets the hydrostatic pressure and pulls fluid into the vascular system.

The blood cells include erythrocytes (red blood cells [RBCs]), leukocytes (white blood cells [WBCs]), and thrombocytes (platelets). These cells primarily originate from hematopoietic (blood cell-producing) stem cells in the bone marrow—for example, in the ribs and the ends of long bones. Stem cells, which exist in both embryonic and adult forms, are primitive cells not only capable of differentiating into other cells, but also of self-replicating to ensure their continuous supply. The hematopoietic stem cells found in the bone marrow are able to differentiate into either myeloid or lymphoid stem cells when specifically stimulated to do so. Lymphoid stem cells are able to produce either T or B lymphocytes, whereas myeloid stem cells can differentiate into RBCs, WBCs, and platelets.

The functions of RBCs include transporting oxygen (O_2) and carbon dioxide (CO_2), and helping maintain acid–base balance. The hemoglobin in RBCs contains heme, an iron compound, and globin, a protein. In the capillaries within the lung, oxygen binds with the iron on this hemoglobin; the oxygen-laden RBCs then flow to body tissues, where the body's cells receive this oxygen supply. Carbon dioxide attaches to the globin protein when CO_2 diffuses from tissue cells into the capillaries; from there, it is carried in the blood to the lungs to be expelled. Hemoglobin buffers excessive acids in venous blood by combining with hydrogen ions, which are produced by cellular metabolism.

Most of the heme found in RBCs is ultimately converted into *bilirubin*, a yellowish or orange-colored pigment in the bile, which is eventually excreted mostly through the feces. Pathologic bilirubin accumulation leads to *jaundice*, which may be evidenced by a yellowish tone of the patient's skin or sclera.

Erythropoiesis (production of RBCs) within the bone marrow is stimulated by erythropoietin, a hormone primarily produced and released by the kidney. This process requires many essential nutrients, including folic acid; vitamins B_{12}, B_2, and B_6; protein; and iron. Destruction of RBCs normally occurs in the bone marrow, liver, and spleen after approximately 120 days—the RBC's average life span.

Thrombocytes (platelets) function primarily to promote blood coagulation by initiating the formation of a platelet "plug" and the clotting process. This series of events can close an opening in the capillary wall to stop bleeding.

Leukocytes (WBCs) play an important role in the body's defensive and reparative mechanism. Granulocytes—that is, WBCs with granules in their cytoplasm—include neutrophils, eosinophils, basophils, and band cells (less mature granulocytes, the presence of which increases in infection). Eosinophils and basophils are said to be involved in hypersensitivity or allergic reactions. Agranulocytes—that is, WBCs without granules in their cytoplasm—include lymphocytes and monocytes.

The two subtypes of lymphocytes are B cells (derived from bone marrow) and T cells (mostly derived from the thymus). B cells provide humoral immunity, whereas T cells provide cell-mediated immunity. Both types of immunity are essential for maintaining human health, though their mechanisms can be complicated. In humoral (antibody-mediated) immunity, antibodies are produced by the B lymphocytes (differentiated B cells) found in plasma (the Greek word *humor* means "body fluid"). Humoral immunity is believed by researchers to need the "help" of T cells in recognizing some antigens and triggering antibody formation. In contrast, in cell-mediated immunity, T cells directly attack antigens—the foreign invaders, such as bacteria or viruses—instead of producing antibodies.

The immune system can be affected by a broad spectrum of factors, including a person's physical or emotional status, diet, or medications; thus, various types of immune system dysfunctions can occur anytime in the course of life. Normally, this system functions primarily to recognize the initial invasion of foreign (non-self) substances, such as microorganisms. It may subsequently develop antibodies and sensitize lymphocytes to mount a specific reaction (the immune response) to ward off repeated invasions of the foreign substance. Over-reaction of the immune system may result in hypersensitivity or allergy. When the ability to accept self-antigen or one's own tissues is impaired, autoimmune disorders may set in.

Immunity may be naturally developed or acquired. Natural immunity involves no prior contact with an antigen. For example, humans are immune to certain infectious agents that cause illness in other species. Acquired immunity can be classified into two types: actively or passively acquired immunity. Actively acquired immunity may develop after a person has a disease or through immunization (i.e., vaccination with a less virulent antigen). Passively acquired immunity develops after a person receives antibodies to an antigen rather than synthesizing antibodies; for example, an infant may obtain antibodies through the mother's breastmilk or through an injection with hepatitis B immune globulin (serum antibodies). Passive immunity is usually short-lived, as it does not lead to the production of memory cells that might offer long-term protection to the individual against future encounters with the antigen.

A blood typing test is usually done before a person donates or receives blood, and for assessing the risk of Rh (Rhesus factor) incompatibility between an expectant mother and her fetus. The ABO blood typing system is based on whether specific blood group antigens (i.e., A and B) are present on RBCs' surface membranes. Group A blood has antigen A and anti-B antibodies, whereas group B blood has antigen B and anti-A antibodies. Group AB blood has both antigens (A and B) and no antibodies to react to the transfused blood; for this reason, individuals with type AB blood are known as universal recipients. Group O blood has neither antigen on its RBCs; individuals with group O blood are known as universal donors because their blood has neither antigen A nor antigen B, but does have both antibodies.

Blood clumping will occur when a patient with the A blood type receives a donor's blood containing B antigens (in either type B or type AB blood), and when a patient with the B blood type receives donated blood containing A antigens. Such a mismatch results in hemolysis of RBCs. Before administering a blood transfusion, it is imperative to confirm that the correct blood type is being given to the correct patient. If a patient who is receiving a blood transfusion starts to feel a vague sense of uneasiness, or have signs or complaints such as nausea, sweating, chills, shortness of breath, or low back pain, the first nursing action is to immediately stop the transfusion and act per protocol; a potential blood type mismatch may be to blame.

The spleen, which is the largest lymphoid organ, is located in the left upper quadrant of the abdomen. It filters the blood and performs many functions, including producing RBCs in the fetus and when bone marrow is damaged in adults, removing old and defective RBCs, recycling iron, filtering circulating bacteria, and storing RBCs and platelets. In addition, the spleen has some immunologic functions, such as forming lymphocytes and monocytes. Nevertheless, this organ is not considered essential to survival.

The spleen is highly vascular. A penetrating injury to it may necessitate a splenectomy to prevent hemorrhage, septicemia, or peritonitis. After a splenectomy, the patient may have immunologic deficiencies; measures should be taken to prevent infection.

DISORDERS AND CONDITIONS

ANEMIA

In anemia, a lower-than-normal hemoglobin concentration is present, reflecting fewer erythrocytes in the blood, which in turn reduces the amount of oxygen delivered to the body tissues. This condition manifests as generalized tissue hypoxia and may be attributable to a host of etiologies. Various terms are used to describe types of anemia based on different etiologies or criteria. Some of the more common types are discussed in this section.

Main Symptoms

Symptoms are influenced by many factors, including the rapidity of development, durations, patients' conditions, and underlying disorders. The tissue hypoxia associated with anemia (due to different causes) commonly accounts for the following manifestations:

- Pallor
- Dyspnea on exertion

- Palpitation
- Dizziness
- Chronic fatigue

Nutritional anemia may result from a deficiency of iron, vitamin B_{12} (cobalamin), or folic acid.

Iron-deficiency anemia may be induced by factors such as inadequate iron intake, malabsorption, excessive loss of iron due to blood loss, or red blood cell trauma. In addition to changes in lab values, such as low hemoglobin levels (because iron is needed for the formation of hemoglobin), other common clinical findings may include the following:

- Fatigue, inability to concentrate, and exertional dyspnea
- Cracks at the corners of the mouth, and inflammation of the tongue (glossitis) or lips (cheilitis)
- Pica (eating non-food) behavior in some cases
- Headache or numbness/tingling in the extremities

In pernicious anemia, a type of megaloblastic anemia (characterized by abnormally large erythrocytes), there is a deficiency of vitamin B_{12} due to various causes—for example, inability to absorb cobalamin or loss of intrinsic factor, which is needed for vitamin B_{12} absorption. Loss of intrinsic factor can result from a partial or total removal of the stomach, as intrinsic factor is produced by mucosal cells in this organ. Patients with pernicious anemia may have a sore tongue, weakness, and paresthesia (numb and tingling sensations in the extremities).

Aplastic anemia may be caused by a depression of the bone marrow or injury to stem cells, resulting in pancytopenia (decreased production of all blood cells—RBCs, WBCs, and platelets). The symptoms vary with the severity of the condition. This type of anemia may be idiopathic (without recognizable cause) or triggered by a specific factor, including chemical agents, toxins, severe disease, or radiation.

In sickle-cell anemia, a genetic disorder, the RBCs tend to assume a sickle shape in response to a low oxygen level. Sickle-cell anemia can be precipitated by hypoxia resulting from stressful conditions such as infection, high altitude, or blood loss. The sickle-shaped cells cannot easily pass through blood capillaries, which leads to blood vessel obstruction, impaired circulation, and anemia. Such cell sickling can result in RBCs destruction (hemolysis); if it is not reversed with sufficient oxygenation in time, serious complications can develop. One of the main symptoms of sickle-cell disease is severe pain due to lack of oxygen in tissues. Chronic sickle-cell anemia may manifest as pallor of the mucous membranes, activity intolerance, swollen joints, and fatigue. Severe oxygen depletion of the tissues and hypovolemia can result in life-threatening shock.

Anemia may also stem from renal disease. When renal function is impaired, the kidneys' production of erythropoietin, which stimulates red blood cell production, will be affected. Notably, patients undergoing dialysis may lose blood into the dialyzer, contributing to iron deficiency and anemia.

Selected Nursing Tips

1. Manage different types of anemia according to their specific nursing guidelines for each. Eliminate identifiable causes and provide vigorous supportive care. Implement energy-saving practices, such as sitting to perform daily tasks. Monitor lab results and report to the practitioner to get any problems addressed.

2. Encourage patients to consume a nutritionally appropriate diet or obtain recommended vitamin replacement to correct nutritional deficiencies and improve their resistance to infection.

3. Watch lab values, including hemoglobin and hematocrit; be alert to signs of infection. Schedule undisturbed rest periods while patients are hospitalized.

4. When caring for patients with iron deficiency:
   - Advise patients to take liquid iron through a straw to avoid staining the teeth. Vitamin C or orange juice can enhance the absorption of iron.
   - Alleviate and manage the side effects of iron supplementation, which include constipation; increase fluid and

dietary fiber intake as appropriate. Inform patients that iron supplements may turn stools dark-colored, which may mask bleeding.

- Offer non-irritating mouthwashes or foods for patients who have a sore mouth or tongue.
- Tell patients to report the side effects of iron supplements, such as nausea, vomiting, or constipation, for possible dose adjustment. In case of an allergic reaction, stop the iron infusion and be prepared to provide supportive treatment at once.
- Z-track administration of iron intramuscular (IM) injections may prevent side effects such as brownish skin discoloration and irritation at the injection sites.
- Advocate for iron-deficiency prevention in susceptible populations. Foods rich in iron include meats (especially organ meats), eggs, beans, green leafy vegetables, and raisins.
- Stress the importance of compliance with iron supplementation therapy, as iron replacement takes time; prevent overdose or overuse of iron supplements.

5. When caring for patients diagnosed with sickle-cell anemia, one of the priorities is to assess their pain level and control pain with prescribed analgesics. Encourage patients in remission to take measures to prevent exacerbation:

- Avoid wearing tight-fitting, restrictive clothing or participating in strenuous exercise.
- Ensure adequate hydration and practice infection prevention.
- Avoid conditions that may induce hypoxia, including cold temperatures, high altitude, and use of medications that produce vasoconstriction. Promote general health and good hygiene practice.

Points to Consider

1. Counsel patients who have had extensive gastric resections or who are on strict vegetarian diets about the importance

of having prescribed vitamin B_{12} supplementation, possibly for life.

2. Folic acid anemia may be related to chronic alcohol use or inadequate dietary intake.

3. In case of aplastic anemia, in which the patient has a decreased bone marrow production of erythrocytes, leukocytes, and platelets, reverse isolation is usually necessary. Patients should prevent infection by avoiding crowds, practice good hygiene, and eliminate raw foods from their diets.

Precaution

In case blood transfusions are indicated, carefully follow nursing guidelines regarding the proper techniques and policies. Closely monitor the patient for signs of a transfusion reaction, including the highly dangerous acute hemolytic reaction, such as elevated temperature, chills, rash, hives, itching, back pain, or restlessness, which often occur in the initial period of therapy. If allergic reaction is suspected, stop the transfusion immediately.

DISSEMINATED INTRAVASCULAR COAGULATION

Disseminated intravascular coagulation (DIC) may be precipitated by sepsis, cancer, shock, toxins, allergic reaction, or other serious disorders. It is a sign of a serious, potentially life-threatening health problem. The profuse bleeding may be attributed to a variety of factors, including depletion of platelets and clotting factors when excessive amounts of clots are formed in the microcirculation (i.e., platelets and clotting factors get used up in clotting process).

Main Symptoms

Abnormal bleeding into the skin (e.g., petechiae or ecchymosis) may be noted in susceptible patients without a hemorrhagic disorder. Bleeding from an invasive procedure sites, mucous membranes, and the gastrointestinal (GI) or urinary tract may also occur. Patients may have abnormal lab results, including progressively decreasing platelets, low fibrinogen level, and altered coagulation time, possibly with accompanying signs of serious complications, such as severe muscle pain, cyanosis, dyspnea, or shock.

Selected Nursing Tips

1. To resolve DIC, the underlying conditions must be treated concurrently.
2. Monitor vital signs and blood studies, including hematocrit, hemoglobin, and coagulation test results.
3. Avoid injuries, straining, and rubbing of bleeding areas; use pressure, cold compresses, or prescribed hemostatic agents to stop bleeding.
4. Watch for signs of GI bleeding and shock. Measuring waist girth may be a way to detect the abdominal distension resulting from internal bleeding.
5. Manage fluid and electrolyte balance. When blood transfusion is ordered, carefully adhere to administration guidelines and specifications and closely watch for signs of transfusion reaction or fluid overload.

Point to Consider

New interpretations or theories regarding the pathology of DIC are likely to lead to new treatment approaches.

Precaution

Prompt recognition and treatment of underlying causal condition are of great significance; caution should be taken to avoid injuries and any precipitating cause of bleeding.

HEMOPHILIA

Hemophilia, a genetically transmitted blood disorder, is characterized by the lack of normal clotting factor VIII (in hemophilia A) or clotting factor IX (in hemophilia B or Christmas disease). This deficiency results in prolonged coagulation time and abnormal bleeding.

Main Symptoms

The severity of this bleeding disorder depends on the degree of clotting factor deficiency and the site of bleeding, with the most dangerous site being in the head:

- In minor cases, patients may present with prolonged bleeding only after major trauma.
- In severe hemophilia, spontaneous or excessive bleeding after minor trauma may cause hematoma. Bleeding into various body parts, especially the joints, may produce pain and disabling effects. Internal bleeding from the urinary or GI tract may also occur.

Selected Nursing Tips

1. Provide therapy as prescribed; treatment may prevent crippling consequences and prolong the patient's life expectancy.
2. Medications with an anticoagulant effect, such as aspirin, should be avoided.
3. Take measures to prevent bleeding, including adopting healthful practices to avoid preventable surgery or procedures, such as ensuring good dental hygiene to avoid tooth extraction.
4. Ensure the safety of the patient's living environment; remove clutter to prevent falls or injuries.
5. Refer the patient and family to genetic counseling when reproductive concerns are an issue.

Point to Consider

Most patients with hemophilia are males. Carriers are females, who may need genetic counseling regarding reproductive concerns.

Precaution

Advise patients to prevent injuries and report signs of internal bleeding, such as blood in the urine and blackish stools.

HUMAN IMMUNODEFICIENCY VIRUS INFECTION

In human immunodeficiency virus (HIV) infection/acquired immunodeficiency syndrome (AIDS), the patient's immune system is severely compromised. HIV is transmitted by direct contact with infected blood or body fluids. It is not spread through casual social contact, such as hugging or dry kissing.

Medical terms that are frequently used in caring for patients with HIV or AIDS include *viral load*, meaning the number of the viral particles in the plasma (measured via a test), and *CD4+ T-cell count*, whose decline may be indicative of an impaired immune system.

HIV infects human cells that have CD4 receptors on their surfaces, especially T cells. T cells, which are also known as T-helper cells or CD4+ T-lymphocyte cells, are believed to have more CD4 receptors on their surface than other cells also bearing CD4 receptors.

CD4+ T cells play a key role in recognizing and fighting pathogens. When they are infected and destroyed, and if the body is unable to produce enough new CD4+ T cells to replace the destroyed cells, immune function will be compromised. When HIV-positive patients have a low CD4+ T-cell count, they may develop severe health problems. HIV infection may progress to AIDS—a condition in which patients develop opportunistic diseases, such as oral candidiasis or Kaposi's sarcoma.

Main Symptoms

The disease process and manifestations of HIV/AIDS are largely individualized and not usually predictable. When initially infected with HIV, patients may experience a flu-like illness characterized by symptoms including fever, sore throat, malaise, diarrhea, and rash. Patients may then be able to maintain a level of CD4+ T-cell count for many years with only vague and nonspecific symptoms. When the CD4+ level drops further, patients may develop worsening symptoms, such as persistent fever, drenching night sweats, and chronic diarrhea.

Candidiasis or thrush, herpes, bacterial infections, shingles, and Kaposi's sarcoma can also occur.

Patients with AIDS who develop *Pneumocystis jiroveci* (formerly known as *Pneumocystis carinii*) pneumonia (PCP) are often acutely ill. The increased metabolism associated with PCP can cause sweating, diarrhea, vomiting, fever, tachypnea, tachycardia, and other manifestations.

Selected Nursing Tips

1. Evaluating the pattern of CD4 cell counts over time is more important than any single test result to assess the effectiveness of antiviral therapy, along with viral load testing (which measures the quantity of HIV particles in the blood).
2. Provide education and counseling regarding the risk factors and preventive methods, including abstaining from sharing body fluids or drug needles in any way.
3. When caring for patients during the terminal phase of AIDS, provide palliative care to keep them comfortable, maintain a restful environment, encourage expression of concerns, and enhance coping mechanisms.

Points to Consider

1. Screening for HIV antibodies has minimized the risk of AIDS transmission associated with blood transfusions. While there is still a "window period" following exposure to the virus during which HIV antibodies may not be detectable, the risk that blood donations from infected individuals will be mistakenly accepted has been minimized or eliminated through many screening and preventive measures.
2. *Pneumocystis jiroveci* pneumonia is an opportunistic lung infection, often seen in immunocompromised individuals, including patients who have HIV infection, leukemia, or lymphoma, and those who have undergone organ transplantation. Treatment outcomes for this infection have considerably improved in recent years, thanks to continuing research.

3. HIV treatment protocols are frequently updated; the new therapies and drugs available for patients have improved their life quality and expectancy.

Precautions

1. Patients' strict adherence to drug regimens is especially important with HIV/AIDS because missing even a few doses of prescribed drugs can lead to viral mutations, resulting in HIV becoming resistant to the drugs.
2. Practicing universal and standard precautions is key to HIV infection prevention.

LEUKEMIA, RELATED TO

In leukemia, a hematologic malignancy, the rapid turnover of blood cells affects the bone marrow, leading to decreased production of normal blood cells. This deficiency eventually affects the patient's major organs, such as the liver and spleen. Leukemia can strike people of all age groups.

Various terms are used to describe leukemia based on the type of white blood cell involved and specific criteria or characteristics, including acute (or chronic) lymphocytic leukemia and acute (or chronic) myeloid leukemia.

Main Symptoms

Symptoms vary depending on the types or stages of disease. Generally, patients with leukemia may experience the following signs and symptoms:

- Fever and infection (because of a lack of sufficient mature white blood cells to defend against infection)
- Fatigue, weakness, and pallor
- Palpitation, tachycardia, and dyspnea
- Signs of hematologic disorders, such as anemia or abnormal bleeding (e.g., nosebleed, easy bruising)

Selected Nursing Tips

1. Provide prescribed treatment therapy to achieve the longest possible periods of remission (e.g., medication, platelet or red blood cell transfusion, or even bone marrow or stem cell transplant in some cases), relieve symptoms, and prevent infection.
2. Promote good nutrition, adequate fluid intake, and general comfort. Minimize constipation and the adverse effects of treatment, such as chemotherapy, and prevent complications.
3. Practice reverse isolation: Protect the patient from being exposed to infections or communicable diseases.
4. Ensure safety and prevent injuries. For example, patients should avoid using bladed or other sharp tools to prevent injuries and bleeding. Applying pressure or a cold pack to a bleeding area or elevating an injured limb, as appropriate, may help stop bleeding.

Points to Consider

1. Dietary counseling may be needed, as some medications can alter the nutritional status of patients with leukemia.
2. It is generally advisable for patients with leukemia to avoid raw fruits or vegetables and undercooked food.

Precaution

Monitor the patient for early signs of infection (e.g., elevated temperature, cough, sore throat) or abnormal bleeding (e.g., bruising, ecchymosis), and initiate treatment promptly as indicated.

LYMPHOMA

Lymphoma, a malignancy of the cells of lymphoid origin, may be generally termed as Hodgkin and non-Hodgkin. The exact cause of this malignancy is unknown.

Hodgkin Lymphoma

In Hodgkin (or Hodgkin's) lymphoma, the malignant cells known as Reed–Sternberg cells are characteristically present. The cause of their development remains unknown. Proper, timely treatment of Hodgkin lymphoma can increase survival rate; this disease is now potentially curable owing to advances made in therapy.

Main Symptoms

The first sign of Hodgkin lymphoma may be painless enlargement of one or more lymph nodes. Manifestations of the disease may involve multiple systems depending on the disease stage, including generalized itching, B symptoms (e.g., fever, night sweats, and weight loss), dyspnea, and malaise. Systemic involvement eventually affects the major organs, such as the spleen, liver, and bones. In the late stage, other features of Hodgkin lymphoma may include edema, anemia, and susceptibility to infection.

Selected Nursing Tips

1. Provide treatments aiming for a cure and manage problems related to the disease or the side effects of therapy (e.g., chemotherapy and/or radiation therapy).
2. Provide small, frequent meals with sufficient nutrition and adequate fluids to improve general health, so as to stave off infection.
3. The skin in the radiation field requires special nursing attention to prevent complications; keep skin in radiated areas dry and free from irritation.
4. Promote the patient's self-care and disease management abilities, stressing the importance of preventing second malignancies by reducing risks, including use of tobacco or alcohol, exposure to excessive sunlight, and exposure to other environmental carcinogens.

Points to Consider

1. The large, unique Reed–Sternberg cell is the hallmark of Hodgkin lymphoma; its presence may be revealed via one or more biopsies.
2. With advanced therapy, Hodgkin lymphoma is potentially curable—a fact that may be shared with patients, if appropriate, to encourage a positive outlook and compliance with treatment.

3. Refer the patient and family to local services for supportive assistance wherever available.

Precaution

Minimize the pain and bleeding associated with stomatitis (inflammation of the mouth) resulting from therapy by using a soft toothbrush and proper cleansing agents (e.g., alcohol-free mouthwash).

Non-Hodgkin Lymphoma

A considerable number of subtypes of lymphoma originating in the lymphoid tissues are not defined or diagnosed as Hodgkin lymphoma; instead, they are known as non-Hodgkin lymphoma (NHL). In NHL, the lymphoid tissues are often infiltrated by cancer cells and the disease is frequently not localized.

Main Symptoms

The symptoms of NHL vary widely, and the patterns of spread are unpredictable or erratic, reflecting the disease's variable nature. It sometimes presents with a painless lymph node enlargement, accompanied with other manifestations depending on the locations to which the NHL has spread.

NHL can involve different systems. By the time it is diagnosed, the patient may display symptoms specific to the areas involved. Patients may also complain of fatigue and have B syndromes (fever, night sweat, malaise, and unintended weight loss).

Selected Nursing Tips

1. Based on the stage of disease and affected body systems, manage symptoms stemming from NHL, such as pain related to tumor, pancytopenia, and adverse effects of the treatment.
2. Counsel patients about strategies to alleviate or cope with systemic side effects of chemotherapy, including nausea, hair loss, infection susceptibility, and side effects arising from the areas being radiated (e.g., skin irritation).
3. Implement energy-saving practices to lessen fatigue, which is generally experienced by patients receiving either chemotherapy or radiation therapy.

4. Listen to the concerns of patients and their families and provide emotional support as appropriate.

Point to Consider

The treatment of NHL is often not as effective as the treatment of Hodgkin lymphoma because chemotherapy is more effective in treating faster-growing cells.

Precaution

Patients need to be reminded to minimize their risks of infection and report early signs due to the nature of the condition and its therapy.

MULTIPLE MYELOMA

In multiple myeloma, a malignancy affects the marrow plasma cells that secrete immunoglobulins (proteins necessary for the production of the antibodies that combat infections). The result is an increase in the volume of nonfunctional immunoglobulins, which often infiltrate or otherwise affect the bones and other organ tissue. When the production of normal red blood cells, white blood cells, and platelets is disrupted, patients may experience problems stemming from anemia, episodes of infection, bone destruction, and soft-tissue or organ damage. Factors potentially influencing a person's risk of developing this type of plasma cell cancer include exposure to radiation, chemicals, or viral infection.

Main Symptoms

- Bone pain, often in the back and ribs
- Arthritic symptoms, such as joint swelling and achiness, and possible pathologic fractures or vertebral compression
- Anemia and increased susceptibility to infection due to impaired production of the blood cells and antibodies
- Hypercalcemia (high blood calcium level), as calcium is released from bone destruction, with patients subsequently

displaying signs such as confusion, polyuria, GI problems, or seizure
- Fever, peripheral paresthesia, or malaise

The M (monoclonal) protein produced by the myeloma cells may be detected in urine and blood tests.

Selected Nursing Tips

1. Relieve bone pain and minimize the side effects of medications (e.g., nonsteroidal anti-inflammatory drugs [NSAIDs]), such as GI distress.
2. Ensure the patient's adequate hydration, and monitor fluid intake and output.
3. Assist the patient to walk and be mobile, as immobilization increases bone demineralization and leaves the patient more vulnerable to complications. If the patient is bedridden, maintain good alignment, do passive range-of-motion exercise, and log-roll the patient when turning him or her.
4. Encourage the patient to engage in safe exercise as tolerated to promote lung expansion. Some activity restriction may be necessary to prevent fractures.
5. Alleviate adverse effects of chemotherapy or radiation therapy. Observe for signs of infection or fracture, such as fever, malaise, or pain. Note that steroidal medications may mask the signs of infection.

Points to Consider

1. Weight-bearing activities such as walking promote bone reabsorption of calcium.
2. Adequate fluid intake may dilute the blood and prevent renal complications, resulting from renal tubular obstruction due to the presence of large amounts of abnormal protein, hypercalcemia, and hyperuricemia.
3. Analgesics should be taken as ordered or before pain becomes too severe.

Precaution

Provide a walker and support the patient as necessary to prevent falls, as individuals with multiple myeloma are prone to fractures.

SYSTEMIC LUPUS ERYTHEMATOSUS

Systemic lupus erythematosus (SLE) is characterized by an abnormal immune regulation that results in excessive production of autoantibodies. Multiple body systems can be affected in lupus, a complex inflammatory disease of the connective tissues. The exact cause of SLE is unclear, but there is evidence suggesting interaction of many factors, including genetic, hormonal, and immunologic involvement. Environmental hazards (e.g., sunlight or thermal burns) and certain medications have also been implicated in inducing this condition. The course of SLE is unpredictable, often marked by remissions and exacerbations. Its severity and manifestations vary widely.

An infection or stressful event can exacerbate SLE. Sun exposure may significantly aggravate the condition.

Main Symptoms

- Erythematous (red) rashes across the nose and cheeks; skin lesions exacerbated by sunlight or artificial ultraviolet (UV) light
- Cardiopulmonary or renal abnormalities, including hypertension
- A wide range of neurologic dysfunction, from subtle personality changes to deterioration in cognitive ability

Selected Nursing Tips

1. Relieve symptoms and manage acute and chronic problems involving affected systems and the side effects of the treatment. Adequate rest, optimal nutrition, and regular exercise may boost patients' immune function and help prevent serious complications.

2. Instruct patients on how to avoid provoking factors. For example, provide skin management tips, such as the use of sunscreen, an umbrella, protective long-sleeved clothing, or a large-brimmed hat to avoid UV/sunlight exposure.

3. Encourage patients to engage in activities that promote general health status. Patients may also benefit from participating in support groups.

4. Counsel patients regarding medication regimens. For instance, explain that topical or oral steroidal medications need to be tapered off before their complete discontinuation with physician's approval. Advise patients on steroid therapy to avoid exposure to acute infection, such as chickenpox or measles.

5. Consult with a dietician and make dietary recommendations pertaining to patients' specific conditions, such as hypertension.

6. Remind patients of the importance of routine follow-ups to assess the effectiveness of treatment and of reporting signs of developing cardiovascular, renal, or neurologic complications.

Points to Consider

1. The ANA (antinuclear antibody) test may be positive in patients with active cases of SLE.

2. NSAIDs may be used in an effort to minimize the corticosteroid medications prescribed for exacerbations.

3. In some cases, only the skin is affected, but the disease may evolve to impact other systems.

Precaution

Take measures to avoid exposure to sunlight and other aggravating factors, such as stress or infection. Prevent calcium and vitamin D deficiencies, which may result from lack of sunlight exposure or dietary inadequacy.

CHAPTER 2

Cardiovascular Issues

The heart is a hollow muscular organ with four chambers. Roughly the size of a fist, the heart consists of three layers of tissues:

- The endocardium (inner lining)
- The myocardium (muscular middle layer)
- The epicardium (fibrous outer layer)

The two-layer pericardium, which resembles a membranous fibroserous sac, houses the heart. Between the two layers of the pericardium is the pericardial space, which normally contains a small amount of serous fluid; this fluid reduces the friction created by the heart's movement.

The heart is vertically separated by the septum. Between the right atrium and the right ventricle is the tricuspid valve; between the left atrium and the left ventricle is the mitral valve. The right atrium takes in venous blood from the inferior and superior venae cavae and the coronary sinus. This blood flows through the tricuspid valve into the right ventricle, which pumps blood through the pulmonic valve into the pulmonary artery and to the lungs with each contraction. (All the arteries transport blood away from the heart. The pulmonary artery is unique in that it is the only artery that carries deoxygenated blood.)

Gas exchange takes place in the lungs between the alveoli and the pulmonary capillaries. Inhaled oxygen diffuses into the capillaries from the alveoli, whereas carbon dioxide diffuses from the blood into the alveoli to be exhaled out of the body.

Oxygenated blood from the lungs enters the left atrium via the pulmonary veins. (All the veins transport blood toward the heart. The blood in the pulmonary veins is oxygenated, unlike that in any other veins.) The bright red blood then runs through the mitral valve into the left ventricle. Once there, it is forcefully ejected by the left ventricle through the aortic valve into the aorta and into high-pressure systemic circulation to meet the needs of the rest of the body cells. Both atria in the heart contract and relax simultaneously, as do both ventricles.

The two coronary arteries (left and right) and their branches supply blood to the heart. Normally there is adequate diastolic (heart relaxing and blood filling) time for myocardial perfusion. However, when the heart rate increases with shortened diastolic time, the blood supply to the heart may not be adequate, especially in patients with coronary artery disease.

DISORDERS AND CONDITIONS

ABDOMINAL ANEURYSM

An aneurysm—that is, an abnormal dilation or outpouching of a weakened site of a blood vessel—often involves an artery. The abdominal aorta is a common site of aneurysms, possibly due to the high volume of blood flow in that area. A variety of factors may be implicated in the development of an abdominal aortic aneurysm (AAA), including smoking, male gender, hypertension, trauma, infection, genetic predisposition, and degeneration.

Degenerative changes due to plaque formation of fatty deposits over the years are likely to result in arteriosclerosis (arterial thickening and hardening) or atherosclerosis (a form of local arteriosclerosis). These conditions are thought to be linked to the loss of elasticity and weakening of the arterial walls, potentially leading to aortic dilation. The larger the size of the aneurysm, the higher the risk of rupture.

Main Symptoms

Most patients with an AAA experience no symptoms. In some patients, a pulsating mass in the area around the umbilicus may be evident with bruits (vascular sounds), which can often be auscultated if the patient is not obese.

If a patient with an AAA experiences a sudden onset of abdominal pain radiating to the lower back and groin, with a numbing or tingling sensation in the feet, and shows signs of hypotension or shock, the impending rupture of the aneurysm may be suspected. Such a rupture is a life-threatening emergency.

Selected Nursing Tips

1. Early detection and prompt treatment are essential to prevent aneurysm rupture and subsequent massive hemorrhage.
2. Be vigilant for signs of rupture, which can be instantly fatal. Signs of acute blood loss include hypotension, tachycardia (rapid heartbeat), tachypnea (rapid respiration), restlessness, and cool and clammy skin. In some aneurysm-rupture cases, the signs of hemorrhage may be subtle, emerging over a period of hours.
3. Once an aneurysm is located, the size should be monitored and any coexisting conditions treated. Reduce the modifiable risks, such as by normalizing blood pressure (BP).
4. Avoid deep palpation, which could rupture the aneurysm.
5. Surgical repair is commonly indicated for a symptomatic patient and a ruptured aneurysm; preparing the patient for surgery may be a nursing priority.
6. After surgery, nursing care aims at maintaining the patient's hemodynamic status to prevent complications. Monitor

pulmonary and renal functions as well as vital signs and lab test results.

Points to Consider

1. A healthy lifestyle, including regular exercise and weight reduction with consumption of a low-fat and low-cholesterol diet, may lower the risk for aortic aneurysm.
2. Male individuals and smokers are more susceptible to abdominal aortic aneurysm of atherosclerotic origin.
3. Ultrasound may be utilized to screen for abdominal aortic aneurysms and to monitor the size of aneurysms.
4. Kidney damage may result when the blood supply is compromised due to shock or repair surgery. Monitor blood urea nitrogen (BUN), creatinine levels, and urine output; urine output of less than 30 mL/h warrants nursing intervention.
5. Individuals with hereditary Marfan's syndrome (a premature degeneration of aortic tissue) may have a relatively higher risk for developing aneurysms and may need to avoid certain vigorous (contact) sports.

Precaution

Auscultate the pulsating abdominal mass for bruits (vascular sounds), but avoid deep palpation to lower the risk of bursting the aneurysm.

CARDIOMYOPATHY, DILATED

Cardiomyopathy (CMP) is characterized by structural and functional abnormalities of the heart muscle that cause impaired heart function and eventually reduced cardiac output, which may lead to increased cardiovascular resistance, and sodium and fluid retention. This condition may be described as dilated, hypertrophic (thickening), restrictive, or others based on its pathology and clinical manifestations, with each variation or a combination of them requiring a different treatment approach.

Dilated cardiomyopathy is relatively more common. It may be idiopathic (with no known cause), or may be linked to a number of different conditions, including alcoholism and nutritional deficiency, resulting in myocardial destruction. The prognosis may vary widely. In dilated cardiomyopathy, ventricle dilatation may affect the heart's ability to eject blood, consequently causing an increased amount of blood to accumulate in the left ventricle after systole contraction.

Main Symptoms

Patients with dilated cardiomyopathy may eventually exhibit signs and symptoms of heart failure (HF): both left-sided failure with respiratory problems (e.g., dry cough, exertional dyspnea, or fatigue) and right-sided heart failure with symptoms (e.g., peripheral edema and jugular vein distension). Other cardiac abnormalities—for instance, dysrhythmias—may also occur in some patients with serious consequences, including sudden death.

Selected Nursing Tips

1. Cardiomyopathy is a life-threatening disorder. Nursing interventions focus on correcting the underlying causes in secondary cases (e.g., controlling heart failure, treating dysrhythmia, maintaining fluid and electrolyte balance, and using diet/lifestyle modifications and palliative measures as appropriate). Early treatment may help minimize the significance of the symptoms and delay the disease process.
2. Record patients' weight on a daily basis to detect fluid retention, which is a sign of heart failure. Ask patients how many pillows are needed to sleep, to help assess for the degree of dyspnea.
3. Warn patients against overexertion or participating in strenuous activities, such as running and lifting heavy objects. Patients should pace their activities to reduce the workload of the heart.
4. Encourage patients to express their feelings, and monitor for signs of depression.

Points to Consider

1. In myocardial hypertrophy, the heart muscle thickening (frequently asymmetrical, particularly along the septum) may affect ventricular filling and eventually reduce the effectiveness of myocardial contractions, potentially increasing the risk of dysrhythmias, such as ventricular tachycardia or ventricular fibrillation. Family members or caregivers may need to learn cardiopulmonary resuscitation (CPR), as sudden cardiac arrest—especially after strenuous physical activity—is possible.

2. In restrictive cardiomyopathy, ventricular filling and stretching may be impaired due to the rigidity of the ventricular walls. In addition, myocardial contractions may be incomplete, reducing cardiac output. Palliative therapy may ease these possible symptoms of heart failure when indicated.

3. When heart failure progresses and other medical-management approaches fail, heart transplantation may be an option for some patients.

4. Sitting with the legs in a dependent position at times may aid in pooling venous blood in the lower extremities and reducing venous return.

Precautions

1. Patients should plan their daily schedule to alternate rest with activity periods so as to prevent overexertion. It is important that patients, especially those with hypertrophic or restrictive cardiomyopathy, avoid strenuous exercise or activities.

2. Medications should be taken as prescribed to maintain therapeutic drug levels and preserve adequate cardiac output.

CORONARY ARTERY DISEASE

Coronary artery disease (CAD) is usually associated with a progressive narrowing of one or more coronary arteries, often due to atherosclerotic plaque buildup. This plaque is formed from deposits of cholesterol, fat, and other blood components. When it obstructs the coronary arteries, the decreased blood flow in turn reduces the oxygen and nutrient supply to the myocardium.

Main Symptoms

Patients with CAD may be asymptomatic. If CAD develops over a long period, the individual may potentially develop collateral circulation to provide the blood supply needed under the normal circumstances.

Some women may not experience the same symptoms typically experienced by men, such as chest pain/pressure, palpitation, or dyspnea. Instead, female patients may have nonspecific symptoms such as fatigue, gastrointestinal (GI) discomfort, or shortness of breath.

Angina or angina pectoris (chest tightness/pain) is one of the main symptoms of CAD. It occurs when myocardial demand for oxygen exceeds the oxygen supply, resulting from inadequate blood flow to the coronary arteries and tissue hypoxia (deficiency of oxygen in body tissues). The pain may be caused by lactic acid buildup due to inadequate tissue oxygenation and anaerobic metabolism. This reversible cardiac muscle ischemia (insufficient blood supply) may follow certain patterns:

- Stable angina is often induced by a predictable amount of exertion or stress.
- Unpredictable angina occurs with increasing frequency, duration, and severity. Over time, it occurs with decreasing levels of stress, even when the patient is at rest. In some patients, this angina may lead to myocardial infarction.
- Prinzmetal's (variant) angina is an atypical form of angina, frequently caused by coronary artery spasm without identifiable triggers. The pain may be experienced at the same time, even at rest.

Severe and prolonged angina may suggest or lead to myocardial infarction. Tissue hypoxia may cause chest pain, possibly accompanied by vomiting, sweating, cool extremities, or fainting.

Selected Nursing Tips

1. Therapy may be geared toward reversing the ischemia by either decreasing myocardial oxygen demand or enhancing oxygen supply. Teach patients strategies to manage acute angina pain, reduce modifiable risks, and minimize precipitating factors, such as physical exertion or stress.

2. Advise patients experiencing pain to stop the triggering activity and to sit down or rest. Nitroglycerin (Nitrostat), a coronary vasodilator, improves blood flow by dilating the blood vessels and reduces cardiac workload. The patient should lie down after placing a nitroglycerin tablet under his or her tongue as directed, because this medication may lower blood pressure and cause dizziness.

3. Sublingual nitroglycerin takes effect in 1–3 minutes. Follow the prescribed administration details; take steps per the protocol (e.g., call for an ambulance) if the patient's pain is not reduced 5 minutes after taking a tablet. It is important to seek emergency medical care in time to rule out myocardial infarction.

4. Advise patients with angina to identify the factors that provoke pain. They should avoid exertion or stress, including strenuous exercise, lifting, straining, emotional upset, and eating heavy meals—all of which increase oxygen demand.

5. During the episode, monitor the patient's vital signs and obtain an ECG or EKG (electrocardiogram), if feasible.

6. Educate patients to reduce modifiable risks:
   - Maintain an optimal serum lipid profile with regular aerobic exercise (or drugs if prescribed) as well as a diet low in fat and cholesterol and high in soluble fibers, which may enhance the removal of cholesterol.
   - Normalize blood pressure.
   - Correct obesity and stop smoking if at all possible.

Points to Consider

1. Certain conditions, including hypertension, diabetes mellitus, and tobacco use, are believed to contribute to vessel injuries and the development of CAD. An elevated level of C-reactive protein (CRP), a nonspecific inflammation marker, or homocysteine, which is formed during the metabolism of an amino acid (methionine), might also play a role in increasing the risk for CAD. (Elevated homocysteine level can also be linked to vitamin B_{12}, vitamin B_6, or folate deficiencies.)

2. Assess the patient's pulse deficit to evaluate the stroke volume when a patient with CAD complains of palpitation. An apical rate greater than the radial rate can be an indication of a possibly inadequate stroke volume (SV) and insufficient cardiac output (COP). A change in either stroke volume or heart rate can affect cardiac output.

3. A cardiac (exercise) stress testing is conducted using an electrocardiograph (EKG) to evaluate the heart's ability to meet increasing oxygen demands. The patient is instructed not to eat for several hours before such a test to prevent aspiration in case of emergency, and to prevent inaccurate results due to blood being diverted from the heart to the stomach for digestion.

4. Over time, walking and exercise can benefit patients with CAD by building collateral circulation, which provides a means of supplying blood around narrowed arteries. (Cardiac events may be more deadly in young patients due to the lack of such collateral circulation.) Exercising in cold weather, however, may cause vasoconstriction, affecting oxygen supply to the heart muscle.

5. Cholesterol, a lipid molecule, is found in both cell membranes and bile. It is also a precursor to steroid hormones. A lipoprotein (or lipid) profile is a blood test that measures several components of the blood to assess the risk of coronary and vascular disease. Low-density lipoprotein (LDL)

cholesterol is also called "bad cholesterol" because it carries cholesterol from the liver to the body cells and can build up on the arterial walls. Conversely, high-density lipoprotein (HDL) cholesterol is often referred to as "good cholesterol" because it carries cholesterol from the body tissues back to the liver, thereby reversing cholesterol transport. Triglycerides, a type of fat carried in the blood, may be associated with the development of atherosclerosis.

6. Some invasive procedures, such as percutaneous transluminal coronary angioplasty (PTCA), traditional coronary artery bypass graft (CABG), and other new alternatives may be used for patients with severe cases of CAD or other cardiac diseases. Prior education and post-procedure management are important nursing functions. Discharge teaching can start when patients first enter the hospital.

7. Consumption of a large amount of grapefruit juice may interact with the statin medications often prescribed to lower blood cholesterol—such as simvastatin (Zocor), atorvastatin (Lipitor), and lovastatin (Mevacor)—by increasing the serum concentration of these drugs and, consequently, their toxicity. Cholestyramine (Questran) should be taken separately, with increased fiber and fluid intake to prevent constipation.

8. Metoprolol (Lopressor) or atenolol (Tenormin), which are antianginal and antihypertensive agents, may slow heart rate and reduce myocardial oxygen requirement. Follow the administration guidelines for these drugs, including checking the patient's blood pressure and apical pulse immediately before giving the medication.

9. Diltiazem (Cardizem), a calcium-channel blocker, has vasodilation effects, thereby reducing peripheral vascular resistance. Assess the patient's vital signs and monitor the pulse rate for sign of bradycardia (slow heartbeat). Remind the patient to get up from a lying position slowly to minimize the impact of gravity on the vascular system, thereby preventing postural hypotension.

Precautions

1. Nitroglycerin is indicated for angina. However, its vasodilating effect may cause severe headaches when it is used as the initial therapy.
2. Insufficient coronary blood flow, even for a very short period of time, may cause irreversible damage to cardiac cells.

ENDOCARDITIS

Endocarditis is usually associated with inflammation or infection involving the endocardium, heart valves, or a prosthetic valve. It often occurs secondary to other conditions, resulting in growth of vegetative lesions in the involved areas, which could break off and cause embolization.

Main Symptoms

- Signs of infection, such as intermittent fever, weakness, and malaise
- A new or changing cardiac murmur
- Possible peripheral manifestations, such as petechiae (small purplish hemorrhagic spots, which are a sign of blood-clotting abnormality)
- Possible features of infarction or vascular occlusion involving affected systems, manifesting as renal, cerebral, or pulmonary abnormalities

Selected Nursing Tips

1. Obtain the patient's allergy history before administering antibiotics. Administer medications on time to maintain therapeutic drug levels. Assess for elevated temperature, worsening murmur, and other signs of infection.
2. Provide supportive treatments, including relieving fever or aches and ensuring sufficient bed rest and fluid intake.
3. Teach the patient and family about the need for possibly longer-term antibiotic therapy to eradicate infection;

patients may also need prophylactic antibiotics later for certain medical procedures, such as dental work.

4. Monitor the patient for signs of heart failure, such as crackles (auscultated over fluid-filled alveoli), edema, distended neck veins, dyspnea, and tachycardia.

5. Perform gentle and thorough oral care to prevent infectious organisms from getting into the bloodstream through the gums.

Point to Consider

A heart valve replacement carries a risk of endocarditis and thromboembolism due to the presence of a foreign substance within the body. Assess patients for their ability to comply with possible long-term anticoagulant therapy to prevent clot formation.

Precaution

Counsel patients about the signs that may indicate the recurrence of endocarditis or complications involving other systems. Advise patients to report symptoms of recurrence of endocarditis, such as fever, anorexia, and night sweats, and signs of embolization, including hematuria (blood in the urine), pleuritic chest pain (related to breathing), and neurologic abnormalities.

HEART FAILURE

Heart failure—a syndrome characterized by poor tissue perfusion and signs of fluid overload—often occurs when the heart can no longer pump adequately to supply the tissues with the needed oxygen and nutrients after its compensatory mechanism is exhausted. As a result, decreased cardiac output (COP) and myocardial dysfunction may lead to vascular congestion, a condition also known as congestive heart failure (CHF).

Heart failure can be related to problems with heart contraction (systolic dysfunction) or heart filling (diastolic dysfunction), among others, and may occur with or without congestion. The underlying mechanism can be complex.

In heart failure caused by systolic dysfunction, the ventricular contraction may be weakened with decreased cardiac output and ejection fraction; in heart failure caused by diastolic dysfunction, the ventricular filling is inadequate, possibly due to heart muscle being stiff and noncompliant. Heart failure can be associated with a variety of conditions, including myocardial infarction, long-standing hypertension, and coronary artery or other cardiovascular diseases.

The following major factors all affect cardiac output:

- Preload: the volume of blood in the ventricles at the end of diastole (when the heart dilates and fills with blood), which is related to the degree of heart muscle stretch
- Afterload: the resistance the left ventricle has to pump against
- Myocardial contractility: the force with which left ventricular ejection occurs (with systole)
- Heart rate
- Metabolic state

Main Symptoms

The symptoms of heart failure are often related to the side of the heart that fails. In many cases, however, heart failure (due to systolic or diastolic dysfunction) affects both sides of the heart, as each side depends on the adequate function of the other. Left-sided heart failure, involving congestion in the lungs, often presents with the following respiratory problems:

- Crackles of cardiac origin, which do not clear with coughing
- A dry, nonproductive cough
- Shortness of breath, decreased oxygen saturation rate, and signs of inadequate tissue perfusion
- Nocturia (possibly due to improved renal perfusion as a result of reduced cardiac workload during resting period)

Right-sided heart failure may occur secondary to left-sided heart failure, with manifestations of systemic fluid retention (as well as the respiratory symptoms):

- Weight gain
- Oliguria (decreased urine output)
- Hypertension
- Dependent edema, evident in the sacral area in bedridden patients
- Jugular vein distension (JVD), an indication of elevated venous pressure and failure of the heart as a pump

The earliest signs of heart failure may include:

- Increased heart rate (when the sympathetic nervous system is activated by a decrease in cardiac output)
- Fatigue due to decreased blood flow to the vital organs

Selected Nursing Tips

1. Follow cardiac care protocols, which are usually updated on a regular basis depending on new theories, discoveries, or technologies. Perform comprehensive assessments, including taking vital signs, recording weight and fluid intake/output, observing activity tolerance, and assessing the severity of dyspnea by determining how many pillows the patient uses to sleep at night.
2. Alleviating pain and anxiety is important to reduce oxygen consumption. Supplemental oxygen should be given as indicated.
3. An upright position facilitates breathing. Placing a patient with heart failure who is experiencing difficulty breathing in a sitting position first, if possible, can reduce the heart's workload by decreasing the venous return and maximizing lung expansion, thereby decreasing pulmonary congestion. Elevating the patient's legs is not encouraged at this time, because increased venous return can worsen pulmonary congestion.

4. Assess for early signs of pulmonary edema, a common and serious complication of heart failure, such as increased heart rate and crackles. Monitor hemodynamic status; record daily weight, the extent of pitting edema, and abdominal girth.

5. Short-term nursing goals may include improved activity tolerance, such as being able to perform daily self-care routines or walking a short distance without dyspnea or air hunger.

6. Table salt and fluid intake may be restricted to manage fluid retention. If so ordered, the goal is to minimize water retention.

7. If a patient with heart failure suddenly develops severe edema in the lower extremities, reviewing the prior intake/output and weight record may help identify a sudden weight gain. This development may be a tell-tale sign of worsening cardiac functioning, indicating a need to adjust the treatment regimen or medication.

Points to Consider

1. Angiotensin-converting enzyme (ACE) inhibitors, such as enalapril (Vasotec) and lisinopril (Prinivil/Zestril), can lower blood pressure by suppressing the renin-angiotensin-aldosterone system, decreasing secretion of aldosterone, and inhibiting conversion of angiotensin I to angiotensin II (a potent vasoconstrictor). When one of these agents is prescribed for management of heart failure (or for other uses), teach patients the measures to minimize its hypotensive effect. Sitting on the side of the bed and rising slowly before standing may help restore equilibrium and prevent dizziness. If an excessive decrease in blood pressure occurs, to offset the hypotensive effect, have the patient lie supine with the legs elevated, if appropriate.

2. When patients receive beta-adrenergic blockers, such as carvedilol (Coreg), watch for bradycardia as well as

hypotension and dizziness, among other adverse effects. Check blood pressure and apical pulse before administering the medication.

3. Digoxin (Lanoxin) can increase the force of heart contraction and slow the heartbeat. It has a narrow therapeutic range. Before administering digoxin, it is essential to determine the patient's apical pulse rate, which is more accurately assessed with a stethoscope over the heart's apex (the pointed part) at the left fifth intercostal space (space between the ribs) in the midclavicular line. Digoxin should be withheld if pulse is less than 60 per minute, or as per protocol/order.

4. Digoxin toxicity may be manifested by GI upset (e.g., nausea, vomiting, or anorexia), neurologic problems (e.g., headache, weakness, and confusion), or visual disturbances (e.g., seeing greenish-yellow halos). Digoxin immune FAB (DigiFab) is an antidote in potentially life-threatening cases of digoxin toxicity.

Precautions

1. Potassium-depleting diuretics, such as furosemide (Lasix), may cause potassium (and other electrolytes such as sodium or chloride) to be excreted in urine, causing hypokalemia. A patient's complaints of leg cramping and muscle twitching—signs of hypokalemia—should prompt the nurse to check the patient's serum potassium level and report low levels to the practitioner. Potassium, a major intracellular electrolyte, has a significant effect on both skeletal and cardiac muscle activities. Severe hypokalemia can lead to dysrhythmia and cardiac or respiratory arrest. (Hypokalemia may also predispose patients to digoxin toxicity.) Carefully observe the furosemide administration rate (without exceeding it) to prevent acute hypotensive episode and ototoxicity. Supplemental potassium is frequently prescribed along with furosemide. Some foods are naturally rich in potassium, such as bananas, orange juice, and potatoes.

2. Patients on potassium-sparing diuretics, such as spironolactone (Aldactone), should be monitored for signs of hyperkalemia (high potassium level), including GI discomfort, muscle twitching, flaccidity, dysrhythmia, or cardiac arrest, especially when patients already have renal insufficiency. Advise these patients to avoid using a potassium-containing salt substitute.

HYPERTENSION (HIGH BLOOD PRESSURE)

Elevated blood pressure without identifiable causes is also known as essential or idiopathic hypertension (HTN). Secondary HTN can be caused by a variety of conditions, including renal diseases or endocrine disorders, such as pheochromocytoma, hyperaldosteronism, and Cushing's syndrome.

Blood pressure (BP) refers to the pressure of circulating blood against the blood vessel walls. Adequate BP is essential to maintain tissue perfusion. Systolic pressure is the maximum pressure measured when the heart contracts, while diastolic pressure is the lowest pressure measured during ventricle relaxation/filling.

Blood pressure reflects the effects of multiple factors, but especially cardiac output and systemic vascular resistance. Systemic vascular resistance (SVR) is the opposing force of the blood flow/movement within the blood vessels. It is primarily affected by the radius of the arteries and arterioles. Even a small change in the radius will result in a major change in SVR.

Circulatory fluid overload and vasoconstriction (narrowed blood vessels) can both increase BP. In contrast, vasodilators such as nitroglycerin decrease BP.

Main Symptoms

Hypertension is also known as a "silent killer," because patients often demonstrate no symptoms until complications develop. These complications may include vascular changes in major organs, such as the heart, brain, or kidneys, as well as secondary symptoms, such as activity intolerance, angina, and edema.

Selected Nursing Tips

1. In secondary hypertension, therapy is largely directed toward correcting the underlying cause, controlling BP, and lowering risk for complications.
2. Emphasize adherence to the medication regimen, if prescribed, to prevent cardiovascular complications such as stroke or heart attack. Urge patients to monitor their blood pressure at home and report abnormalities as indicated.
3. Encourage lifestyle modifications, including regular exercise, stress reduction, and maintenance of the desired weight.
4. Patients with hypertension should generally avoid food high in salt, as excessive sodium can cause fluid retention via the body's homeostasis mechanism (which keeps electrolytes in balance), thereby increasing both fluid volume and blood pressure.
5. Use the proper cuff size for the patient's upper arm circumference when measuring BP to ensure accurate readings. Obtain BP readings in both arms and in lying or sitting positions for verification when indicated.

Points to Consider

1. The definitive causes of hypertension are not clearly understood. Possible modifiable risk factors include stress, obesity, hyperlipidemia, smoking, and excessive salt intake. Nonmodifiable risk factors include age and genetic predisposition.
2. Uncontrolled hypertension may lead to cardiovascular or renal complications. An extremely elevated blood pressure constitutes a medical emergency. If it is not controlled immediately, serious organ damage can result.

3. While hypertension is common in patients with chronic renal failure (CRF), it can also be the cause of CRF.

4. Follow the nursing protocol and check blood pressure before giving some prescribed medications, such as captopril (Capoten), a vasodilator and antihypertensive agent.

5. Furosemide (Lasix), a diuretic, enhances excretion of sodium, chloride, and potassium, and lowers blood pressure. Watch for its possible adverse effects, including hypokalemia, hyponatremia (low serum sodium level), and dehydration.

Precautions

1. Teach methods to prevent extremely high BP (hypertensive crisis), which, if not lowered immediately, can cause serious damage to major organs. Lowering BP too drastically, however, can compromise cerebral, renal, or coronary perfusion (blood flow).

2. Advise patients who are on antihypertensive agents to rise slowly from a lying position (e.g., dangling the feet on the edge of the bed). A drop in blood pressure due to gravity while changing from a lying position to a standing position may cause postural hypotension, lightheadedness, or even falls.

LEG ULCER: ARTERIAL OCCLUSIVE AND VENOUS STASIS

Leg ulcers are common medical problems. The ulcers caused by peripheral arterial occlusion or venous stasis may have different characteristics.

- Venous leg (stasis) ulcers may result from chronic venous insufficiency, frequently related to inadequate valves in the veins and subsequent swelling with blood pooling in the legs.
- Leg ulcers associated with arteriosclerosis may result from narrowing of the arteries and consequently decreased blood supply to the tissues.

Main Symptoms

Main Differences	Venous Stasis Leg Ulcers	Arterial Occlusive Leg Ulcers
Location	Near medial ankle	Lateral ankle, tips of toes, foot
Skin appearance and characteristics	Brownish; thick, hardened; often warm with dermatitis	Elevation pallor, dependency redness, taut, shiny, cool, dry
Shape	Irregularly shaped	Round, smooth
Pain and itching	Painful ulcer, aching and heaviness in calf or thigh; often itching	Claudication; rest pain in foot; rarely itching
Edema	Lower leg edema	Rare
Capillary refill time	Likely within normal limits (less than 2–3 seconds)	Possibly increased (more than 3 seconds)
Leg elevation	Facilitating venous return	Not encouraged—to allow gravity to promote arterial blood flow

Selected Nursing Tips

1. Suggest preventive measures to patients with venous insufficiency:
   - Promote mobility, ambulation, and exercise.
   - If support stockings are prescribed, they are usually put on before getting out of bed and removed when in bed. Warn patients that stockings, if improperly used, can cause complications.
   - Promote venous return; perform meticulous wound care to prevent infection.
   - Encourage leg elevation if appropriate.

2. Suggest preventive measures to patients with diminished arterial perfusion:
   - Quit smoking if possible.
   - When claudication (calf muscle pain related to walking) or muscle cramping occurs, stop activities and rest to decrease oxygen expenditure and relieve discomfort.
   - Encourage slow walking as tolerated to promote collateral circulation.
   - Participate in regular exercise and rest when pain occurs.
   - Wear comfortable shoes; inspect, clean, and pat dry the feet on a daily basis.
   - Keep the limbs warm; apply lotion to the feet and legs, except in between the toes.

Points to Consider

1. Advocate health-promoting activities. Educate patients that certain habits or behaviors may have a negative impact on peripheral circulation, including smoking, prolonged sitting, crossing legs, wearing restrictive clothing, and immobility.
2. Caution patients with peripheral arterial disease to avoid temperature extremes in the feet, as they may not feel pressure or pain sensations there. Soaking the feet in warm water for a prolonged time may cause skin breakdown. Maintaining a dependent leg position at appropriate intervals of time may facilitate arterial blood flow in the leg and relieve pain.
3. Doppler ultrasound can be used to evaluate the movement of blood and assess the speed of blood flow in large blood vessels in a noninvasive way, providing some information about arterial and venous patency.

Precaution

A nursing intervention is needed when a patient complains of numbness, tingling, or pain in the legs. Such signs of paresthesia signify insufficient blood supply to the extremities.

MYOCARDIAL INFARCTION (HEART ATTACK)

In myocardial infarction (MI), commonly known as a heart attack, part of the heart muscle becomes necrotic due to reduced coronary arterial blood flow. There is only a small window of time before the heart cells start to die after ischemia (a lack of blood supply) takes place. Once infarction (tissue necrosis) occurs, it is not reversible.

When the heart cannot maintain adequate cardiac output due to the loss of functional cardiac muscle, dysrhythmia, cardiogenic shock, or death will ensue if the patient is not treated promptly and effectively.

Different terminologies may be used to describe heart attack based on various sets of criteria. For example, ST-elevation myocardial infarction (STEMI) and non-ST-elevation myocardial infarction (NSTEMI) are different diagnostically and have different underlying causes. In STEMI, there is often significant damage to the heart caused by arterial blockage and impaired cardiac perfusion; the patient needs emergency care in a specialized facility as soon as possible to save the heart muscle. NSTEMI is also a medical emergency requiring possibly complicated diagnostic processes for its definitive treatment.

Main Symptoms

- Persistent squeezing pain, like a heavy weight on the chest, often radiating to the left jaw, shoulder, neck, or arm, and not relieved by rest or nitroglycerin
- Initially increased BP because of the release of catecholamines (norepinephrine and epinephrine) and stimulation of the sympathetic nervous system with vasoconstriction; eventually decreased BP due to reduced cardiac output
- Diaphoresis, ashen/clammy skin, anxiety, restlessness, and dyspnea
- Possible development of fever due to inflammation related to tissue damage
- Nausea or vomiting

Some patients—especially women, elderly people, and persons with diabetes—may have atypical discomfort or nonobvious symptoms, such as weakness or shortness of breath.

Selected Nursing Tips

1. Administer oxygen to patients suspected of having an MI to prevent further damage to the heart muscle. Follow the emergency care protocol; activate the code team or emergency medical system (e.g., call for an ambulance or 911 in the U. S.) as indicated. Work closely with the medical specialists to render timely care to the patient. The therapy may depend on the type of heart attack—for example, STEMI versus NSTEMI. Collaborate with the multidisciplinary healthcare team; take measures to relieve chest pain, stabilize heart rhythm, and reduce myocardial workload. Various medications, percutaneous coronary interventions (PCIs), or other tests and approaches may be used by the team.

2. In managing a life-threatening emergency, follow the most up-to-date emergency care guidelines, protecting the patient from imminent harm and making sure the emergency response system is activated. Observe the specified rules and procedures in rendering emergency medical care, including performing cardiopulmonary resuscitation (CPR) and/or defibrillation as trained or instructed. The ABCD protocol of basic cardiopulmonary resuscitation include employing proper skills and equipment or medical supplies to maintain or open the patent's **a**irway, optimize **b**reathing and **c**irculation, and use a standard **d**efibrillator or automated external defibrillator (AED) as indicated (e.g., for ventricular fibrillation and ventricular tachycardia). Cooperate with the emergency rescue team in implementing other emergency interventions per protocols.

3. When assessing patients complaining of chest pain, it is important to ask them to describe the pain, including its location, intensity, and duration. Note that chest pain of pulmonary origin often intensifies upon breathing in.

4. Be sensitive to patients' emotions. Validating their feelings and giving them support or assistance will offer patients a sense of comfort or safety. Offering false hope to patients is not appropriate.

5. An electrocardiogram (EKG), which records the electrical impulses stimulating the heart to contract, can be used for a variety of purposes, including to detect rate changes and arrhythmias. Be aware that some patients with MI, including young women, may initially present with atypical symptoms such as weakness, fatigue, or dyspnea with possible normal EKGs. "Time is heart muscle" until MI is ruled out.

6. Measurement of the serum level of troponin (a myocardial muscle protein) is often used to assess cardiac muscle injury in patients with suspected acute coronary ischemic syndromes or MI, as troponin is released when cardiac cells are damaged. The troponin level rises sooner and stays elevated longer than many other enzymes specific to cardiac injuries, such as CK-MB (creatinine kinase and myocardial bands).

7. When a patient is on thrombolytic therapy and complains of itching or develops generalized urticaria, stop the infusion first, then act and report accordingly per protocol. Other signs of anaphylactic reaction may include irritability, stridor, dyspnea, and hypotension.

8. An important nursing goal for post-MI patients with decreased cardiac output is to improve activity tolerance with no dyspnea or pain on exertion.

Points to Consider

1. For patients with suspected myocardial infarction, follow the current care recommendations. The patient may be given medications (e.g., aspirin, nitroglycerin) as well as oxygen. If morphine is administered, it may reduce the myocardial oxygen demand, so monitor for this

medication's side effects, including respiratory depression and constipation.

2. Thrombolytic agents—such as alteplase, a tissue plasminogen activator (t-PA)—can dissolve clots in a recently obstructed blood vessel. It is crucial to ascertain the time of the onset of symptoms (optimally within the first 3 hours or per the manufacturer's specified time frame) so as to weigh the benefit of using the thrombolytic medication against the risk of serious bleeding and other side effects. Potential drug interactions or contraindications are another important consideration and should be brought to the physician's attention.

3. A common complication of acute MI is dysrhythmia, as the infarction interrupts cardiac perfusion and impulse conduction; this disruption is often the cause of death. Heart failure can also result from MI due to decreased cardiac output or circulatory congestion. Cardiogenic shock may occur when a large area of the myocardium is affected.

4. The specific use of an anticlotting medication, such as clopidogrel (Plavix), prasugrel, or ticagrelor, may be considered and prescribed by the physician. Observe for signs of adverse effects of the anticoagulant; monitor lab results.

5. Anticoagulants, including aspirin or ibuprofen, are usually withheld for several days prior to surgeries or invasive procedures as per protocol. Monitor patients who are on anticoagulants for signs of bleeding, such as epistaxis (nosebleed), hematuria (blood in the urine), and tarry stools.

6. When protamine sulfate—the antidote for heparin—is used to treat severe heparin overdose, administer it per orders while being careful to prevent serious side effects, including acute hypotension and bradycardia (often due to rapid IV administration). Blood coagulation studies, such as activated coagulation time (ACT) and activated partial thromboplastin time (aPTT), are usually conducted to monitor the effects of heparin therapy.

Precautions

1. Observe the patient for symptoms of fluid retention (e.g., crackles, cough, dyspnea, and edema), which may indicate the development of heart failure. If the patient begins to cough up frothy sputum, complains of a sense of drowning, and has dyspnea and tachycardia, then suspect severe cardiac decompensation and pulmonary edema—a medical emergency.

2. Myocardial infarction can lead to cardiac arrest with an immediate loss of consciousness, pulse, blood pressure, and effective breathing. It is essential to follow the most current emergency protocol and treatment guidelines when MI is suspected. Activate the emergency medical services system or code team; properly use the indicated treatment options, including defibrillation, cardiopulmonary resuscitation (CPR), and emergency drugs per (possibly standing) orders.

3. Severe uncontrolled hypertension (as well as a number of other conditions such as active internal bleeding) is a contraindication to thrombolytic therapy due to the risk of cerebral hemorrhage.

PERICARDITIS

In pericarditis, there is inflammation of the pericardium, the two-layered sac enclosing the heart, which normally contains a small amount of serous fluid to separate the two layers. This condition may be either acute or chronic.

Main Symptoms

The common manifestations of acute pericarditis include the following symptoms:

- Sudden chest pain worsened by inspiration and lying supine
- Pericardial friction rub
- Dyspnea or fever

Chronic pericarditis may be asymptomatic or be associated with signs of gradually developing right-sided heart failure, such as fluid retention.

One of the complications of acute pericarditis is pericardial effusion (excess fluid in the pericardial sac); its symptoms resemble those of heart failure, such as dyspnea or tachycardia as well as a feeling of fullness in the chest. When fluid accumulation occurs rapidly, cardiac tamponade, a life-threatening complication, may result.

Selected Nursing Tips

1. Treat underlying causative problems and relieve symptoms.
2. Provide bed or chair rest and oxygen (as appropriate) when the patient has fever and pain; administer medications as ordered, such as aspirin or ibuprofen (Motrin), to reduce pain and inflammation. Indomethacin (Indocin), which is also a nonsteroidal anti-inflammatory drug (NSAID), is not used for patients with certain conditions, including cardiac dysfunction, due to its side effects. Review the medications the patient is taking and report the concurrent anticoagulant use to the practitioner.
3. Having the patient sit up and lean forward, if possible, may alleviate the pleuritic chest pain associated with pericarditis and facilitate breathing.
4. Monitor the patient with acute pericarditis for signs of complications, including cardiac compression, pericardial effusion, and cardiac tamponade.

Points to Consider

1. Rapid accumulation of even a small amount of fluid in the pericardium may not allow the sac the time needed to stretch, thereby compressing the heart. When the compression affects ventricular filling and pumping, cardiac tamponade—a life-threatening medical emergency—may occur.

2. Steroid medications may produce effective relief of the symptoms of pericarditis, but the symptoms may recur when the therapy is discontinued.

Precaution

Cardiac tamponade requires immediate treatment; have equipment readily available for the anticipated procedures.

RAYNAUD'S DISEASE

Raynaud's disease (a primary condition) is characterized by episodes of vasospasm of the small arteries in the digits, which is evidenced by changes in sensation and color of the tips of the fingers or toes. Episodes may be brought on by vasoconstriction related to cold temperature, emotional upset, or use of nicotine or caffeine. This disease commonly involves the tips of the digits bilaterally, with no apparent underlying conditions.

When the problem of episodic vasospasm is associated with several connective tissue disorders such as rheumatic arthritis and systemic lupus erythematosus with a progressive course, it is often termed Raynaud's phenomenon. It is difficult to differentiate Raynaud's disease from Raynaud's phenomenon because some patients with mild symptoms for several years may later develop connective tissue disorder.

Main Symptoms

Raynaud's disease/phenomenon is characterized by color changes of the fingers, toes, ears, or nose. After exposure to cold or stress, the patient may report feeling numbness or tingling, mainly in the fingers, which exhibit typical color changes (pallor, cyanosis, and redness). These changes are usually reversed by application of warmth.

Selected Nursing Tips

1. Advise the patient to keep the hands warm and to wear protective gloves in cold weather or when handling cold

items. The discomfort caused by vasospasm can often be alleviated by immersing the hands in warm water.

2. The nurse should assess the patient for diminished peripheral pulses associated with this condition.

3. Identify and manage the underlying condition in secondary Raynaud's phenomenon. The initial treatment is often conservative due to the adverse effects of vasodilator drugs, which are reserved to treat intolerable symptoms.

Point to Consider

Advocate smoking cessation, stress reduction, and avoidance of injuries.

Precaution

Some medications with vasoconstrictive effects, including cough and cold preparations containing pseudoephedrine (Sudafed), can aggravate this condition and should be avoided.

RHEUMATIC FEVER/RHEUMATIC HEART DISEASE

Rheumatic fever, an acute systemic inflammatory complication of group A streptococcal infection, occurs mostly during the school years. For example, it may follow the development of acute pharyngitis (sore throat), in which antibodies are thought to be produced and involved. Though rare, rheumatic fever may affect people of any age.

Rheumatic heart disease refers to cardiac complications of rheumatic fever, including myocarditis, pericarditis, endocarditis, and chronic valvular disease.

Main Symptoms

The manifestations of rheumatic fever include the following signs and symptoms:

- Fever
- Joint pain, swelling, or redness

- Transient involuntary movement (chorea)
- Carditis, potentially affecting all layers or the valves of the heart

Severe carditis may lead to heart failure, evidenced by symptoms including dyspnea, tachycardia, a hacking cough (possibly due to pulmonary congestion) and significant heart murmurs.

Selected Nursing Tips

1. Encourage the patient complaining of a sudden sore throat, pain on swallowing, and fever to seek treatment, because streptococcal infection may seem like a common cold.
2. Promote adequate rest in support of medication-based treatment. Weeks of bed rest may be prescribed in the acute phase.
3. Instruct the patient and family to watch for signs of heart involvement or failure, such as dyspnea or hacking cough; promptly report the signs of recurrent streptococcal infection, such as sore throat.
4. Patients with a history of rheumatic fever are susceptible to recurrence of the disease. Explain the need to comply with possibly long-term antibiotic therapy and the need for additional antibiotics, if prescribed, as prophylaxis for invasive procedures, such as dental work.

Point to Consider

Effective management of the symptoms and disease may eradicate streptococcal infection and minimize the chance of recurrence and permanent cardiac damage.

Precaution

Before giving penicillin to a patient, ask about the patient's allergies and warn about possible hypersensitivity reactions. If the patient develops allergy symptoms, such as rash or chills, at any time during penicillin therapy, stop the medication immediately and take appropriate nursing actions.

SHOCK, CARDIOGENIC

Shock is a syndrome characterized by failure of the circulatory system to deliver adequate blood and oxygen supplies to the vital organs. Its etiologies may include hypovolemia, vasodilation, and inadequate cardiac output, singly or in combination. It results in decreased tissue perfusion and impaired cellular metabolism. Depending on its precise etiology, the clinical presentation and treatment approach may vary.

In cardiogenic shock, the heart fails to contract adequately and pump blood effectively, resulting in diminished cardiac output that impairs tissue perfusion. This failure may be attributable to either coronary problems, such as acute myocardial infarction, or noncoronary conditions that stress the myocardium or impair heart function, such as severe hypoxemia, hypoglycemia, end-stage cardiomyopathy, ventricular dysrhythmia, and cardiac tamponade.

When the body's compensatory efforts eventually fail, cardiac output declines even further. In turn, the patient exhibits signs of decompensation.

Main Symptoms

Symptoms of shock vary with the underlying condition. In cardiogenic shock, poor tissue perfusion may produce the following acute and profound symptoms:

- Initial signs such as altered level of consciousness and restlessness due to low cardiac output, which causes inadequate cerebral blood flow and a change in mental status
- Hypotension and decreased urine output
- Tachypnea (increased respiration)
- Tachycardia (rapid heart rate)
- Cold, clammy, cyanotic skin

Selected Nursing Tips

1. A major nursing function is to identify risks in vulnerable patients and take preventive measures to lower them,

including administering supplemental oxygen, relieving angina, correcting fluid and electrolyte imbalances, and reducing energy expenditure.

2. When the patient is having difficulty breathing and cardiogenic shock is suspected, act in accordance with the nursing protocol; activate emergency care system as indicated. Provide adequate oxygenation, and implement emergency procedures and treatments as per orders or protocol. Check the blood pressure and pulse, maintain the patient's airway and venous access, keep the patient warm, and monitor urine output.

3. In a patient with emerging shock, placing the patient in a supine position with the legs elevated may facilitate blood flow to vital organs, improving cerebral perfusion via gravity.

4. Work in collaboration with multidisciplinary healthcare team to restore the patient's cardiac function and prevent shock from progressing. Monitor the patient's cardiac and hemodynamic status, implement nursing interventions and therapies to treat the underlying causes, promote cardiac output, enhance myocardial perfusion, and reduce cardiac workload to maintain a balance between oxygen supply and demand.

5. Monitor the patient's vital signs and lab results. Optimal oxygenation may help correct metabolic acidosis and hypoxia, which may be evidenced by the results of arterial blood gas (ABG) studies.

6. Provide emotional support to the patient and family, and work with other members of the healthcare team to coordinate care.

Points to Consider

1. Anaphylactic shock usually results from an acute hypersensitivity reaction to an antigen (e.g., penicillin, latex, eggs, peanuts) to which the patient has been exposed and sensitized previously and then developed antibodies.

Subsequently, a massive release of vasoactive substances, such as histamines, causes vasodilation and increased capillary permeability, such that fluid leaks into the interstitial space. The patient may experience a wide range of symptoms, including shortness of breath, stridor due to laryngeal edema, and hypotension that progresses to shock. The skin may be flushed and itching (pruritus) may be present, along with the eruption of urticaria (hives or wheals). Prompt medical and nursing interventions are crucial to prevent a hypersensitivity reaction from progressing into anaphylactic shock and circulatory failure.

2. In septic shock, the pathology may be complex, but is often associated with a microorganism. A systemic inflammatory response or an infection may be present, combined with increased capillary permeability and poor tissue perfusion. When the body's compensatory mechanisms fail, organ dysfunction may progress. Managing the care of a patient with sepsis or septic shock requires a concerted effort from the entire healthcare team, in which a nurse can play an important role.

3. Dopamine, a vasopressor and cardiac stimulant (adrenergic agonist), may be used as an adjunct therapy in treating shock associated with MI or other conditions. It can improve cardiac contractility and increase cardiac output. Correct the patient's blood volume depletion before administering this medicine when it is prescribed; continuous cardiac monitoring of the patient is a must. Immediately report significant change in vital signs, decreased urine output, or signs of dysrhythmia or reduced peripheral circulation (e.g., cold, mottled extremities). Monitor the IV infusion closely and watch for signs of extravasation (fluids escaping from a vessel into tissues), which can cause serious tissue damage.

Precautions

1. Monitor and maintain the patient's hemodynamic status, and report critical data immediately.

2. Check the patient first if a sudden change is noted in the telemetry monitor (from normal sinus rhythm to dysrhythmia), and then make sure the EKG electrodes are in the right places as indicated.

(CARDIAC) TAMPONADE

In cardiac tamponade, a rapid increase in intra-pericardial pressure (often resulting from blood or fluid buildup in the pericardial sac) compresses the heart, affecting diastolic filling of the heart, and decreasing cardiac output. This acute condition is a life-threatening medical emergency.

Main Symptoms

The following classic signs indicate the failure of the compensatory mechanism and the reduced stroke volume in cardiac tamponade:

- Distant (muffled) heart sounds
- Narrowed pulse pressure (the difference between the systolic and diastolic pressure readings) due to diminished systolic BP, and paradoxical pulse or a drop in inspiratory systolic BP
- Diaphoresis (profuse sweating) and pale, clammy skin
- Dyspnea and restlessness
- Jugular vein distension (possibly due to the heart's inability to pump the fluid back into the circulation)

Selected Nursing Tips

1. Therapeutic approaches depend on the causes, but are aimed at relieving the intra-pericardial pressure and cardiac compression. Monitor the patient's vital signs and administer oxygen therapy.
2. It is important to have the necessary equipment readily available for possible emergency procedures, including pericardiocentesis, in which a needle is inserted into the pericardial sac to aspirate fluid or blood and thereby relieving the pressure on the heart. Cardiac and hemodynamic

monitoring and careful post-procedural management per guidelines and orders are essential. Monitor the patient closely for signs of possible complications of pericardiocentesis, such as myocardial trauma, pleural injury, and dysrhythmia.

3. If thoracic surgery is indicated, prepare and teach the patient what to expect postoperatively (e.g., chest tube and drainage system) and how to cough, turn, and deep-breathe.

Point to Consider

The expected results of pericardiocentesis for cardiac tamponade include increased BP, clear breath sounds, heart sounds that are not muffled or distant, and the patient's report of immediate relief.

Precaution

Hours after a heart surgery, if the patient's profuse draining in the chest tube stops, the nurse should check for possible obstruction to prevent pleural effusion and cardiac tamponade.

THROMBOANGIITIS OBLITERANS (BUERGER'S DISEASE)

Thromboangiitis obliterans, also known as Buerger's disease, refers to a non-atherosclerotic inflammatory vaso-occlusive disorder primarily involving the upper and lower extremities. Its etiology is commonly related to tobacco use. This disease is recurrent, and is often seen in young male smokers. In severe cases, it may result in ulceration and gangrene.

Main Symptoms

Symptoms may involve the distal blood vessels of the extremities:

- Claudication (cramp-like calf pain, especially while walking, which results from inadequate blood flow to the feet), which is relieved by resting

- Cold sensitivity, resulting in changes of the skin color of the limbs
- Paresthesia (numbing or tingling sensation)

In the advanced stages of the disease, patients may develop ulceration and experience pain while at rest.

Selected Nursing Tips

1. Educate patients regarding possible causative factors; advise them to avoid triggering activities. Advocate abstinence from smoking.
2. Teach patients proper foot care to prevent ulceration and gangrene. Remind them to wear warm socks and well-fitting shoes; inspect their feet daily for signs of skin breakdown that requires early treatment.

Points to Consider

1. Nicotine causes vasoconstriction, which leads to increased blood pressure, arterial spasm, and decreased circulation, especially in the legs. Claudication or leg ulcer can be aggravated by smoking.
2. Currently, there is no specific effective treatment for Buerger's disease; smoking cessation is strongly recommended. If necessary, refer the patient to a self-help group for support related to smoking cessation.

Precaution

Advise the patient to reduce stress and to avoid extreme temperatures and injuries.

VARICOSE VEINS

Varicose veins are dilated tortuous superficial veins, mainly in the legs. Secondary varicose veins include esophageal varices and hemorrhoids.

The exact cause of varicose veins is unknown. Aside from nonmodifiable factors, such as increasing age or female gender, other predisposing risks for this condition include obesity and prolonged standing related to certain occupations.

Main Symptoms

Patients may feel fatigue, aching, and heaviness in the legs. Initially the varicose veins may be tense and palpable. They may enlarge and protrude, becoming markedly visible.

Selected Nursing Tips

1. Advise the patient to change position frequently and to avoid prolonged standing or sitting.
2. Relieve pain by elevating the varicosed extremity as appropriate.
3. To facilitate venous return, patients should participate in regular, appropriate range-of-motion or active exercise, such as walking. They should wear properly applied stockings, if prescribed, and avoid constrictive clothing or prolonged sitting or standing.

Point to Consider

Slow and steady walking promotes the muscle-pumping mechanism, improving venous circulation. Elevating the legs several times each day can improve venous blood return to the heart, prevent venous stasis, and reduce leg heaviness and fatigue.

Precaution

Several treatment options are available for severe cases. If an invasive procedure is used, remind patients to report any unusual sensation in the affected extremity immediately so that providers can check for possible damage to nearby nerves.

VENOUS THROMBOSIS/DEEP VEIN THROMBOSIS

In venous thrombosis, there is formation of a clot (thrombus), which is commonly associated with vein inflammation—hence the term thrombophlebitis. In deep vein thrombosis (DVT), the clot forms in a deep vein.

Several theories have been proposed regarding the etiology or pathology of venous thrombosis, with different criteria being used in each theory (e.g., Wells' criteria). The following three contributing factors are known as Virchow's triad:

- Venous stasis with reduced blood flow due to factors such as prolonged inactivity (e.g., on a long trip or bed rest after surgery)
- Increased clotting tendency due to etiologies including smoking, polycythemia (excessive red blood cells), or malignancy
- Impaired inner lining of the vein possibly caused by trauma, such as IV puncture or fracture

One serious complication of DVT is pulmonary embolism, which occurs when a detached clot travels to the lungs. Signs and symptoms of this complication include dyspnea, pink-tinged sputum, and restlessness.

Main Symptoms

- Unilateral nonpitting edema of an arm or leg
- Mild to moderate pain (often with a sudden onset), redness, and warmth of the affected extremity
- Fever, chills, or malaise

Some patients may not exhibit any overt symptoms.

Selected Nursing Tips

1. The following measures are recommended to prevent DVT in high-risk patients:
   - Encouraging mobility and early ambulation postoperatively
   - Ensuring adequate hydration
   - Initiating active or passive range-of-motion exercises
   - Properly applying right-size anti-embolism (e.g., TED hose) stockings or devices as ordered to avoid complications; anti-embolism stockings should be put on before the patient gets out of bed

2. Follow the prescribed treatment regimen. Traditionally, therapies have included bed rest and elevation of the affected extremity, which are thought to encourage the clot to adhere to the vein wall, thereby preventing pulmonary embolism.

3. Applying a lukewarm moist pack may have a vasodilating effect and promote comfort.

4. Monitor patients who are on anticoagulants for signs of bleeding, such as bruising and black, tarry stools. Practice vigilance and implement bleeding precautions, including using a soft toothbrush or an electric razor.

5. Discharge instructions should include measures to prevent the recurrence of DVT, including avoiding dehydration and prolonged sitting or standing.

Points to Consider

1. Walking or leg movement may reduce the risk for venous clot formation. When a patient at risk for thrombosis takes a long airplane trip or car ride, changing leg position or walking about the area at intervals may prevent blood stagnation and pooling in the lower extremities.

2. The dosage of warfarin (Coumadin) is adjusted frequently based on the patient's international normalized ratio (INR), which is a standard used to interpret prothrombin times (PT). When a patient's INR is outside the target range, a high INR indicates a higher risk of bleeding, whereas a low INR suggests a higher risk of developing a clot. (The PT result indicates how many seconds it takes for the blood to clot; the result is then converted to INR regardless how and where the PT is obtained.)

3. When vitamin K, the antidote for warfarin, is used to treat warfarin overdose, the amount is usually based on the significance of bleeding.

4. Enoxaparin (Lovenox) is an anticoagulant, which does not significantly impact activated partial thromboplastin time (aPTT) or PT.

Precautions

1. Inflammation of a vein with clot formation can be a complication of surgery; watch for signs of thrombophlebitis and avoid compression of the popliteal area.
2. If a patient has a central venous catheter in an upper extremity, monitor this site, as it is also a risk factor for DVT.

CHAPTER 3

Respiratory Issues

The respiratory system is primarily responsible for gas exchange through ventilation and diffusion. Working in concert with the cardiovascular system, which is responsible for perfusion (supplying blood to organ tissues), the respiratory system provides body cells with oxygen (O_2) to generate energy and eliminates carbon dioxide (CO_2), a waste product of cellular metabolism. This gas exchange occurs between the alveoli, the lung's microscopic air sacs, and the capillaries surrounding the alveoli. The gas concentration differences in the alveoli and blood provide a diffusion gradient across the alveolar–capillary membrane, which drives O_2 in and CO_2 out of the lungs.

The upper respiratory tract comprises mainly the nose, sinuses, nasal passage, pharynx, tonsils, epiglottis, adenoids (lymphoid tissues), larynx, and trachea. The lower respiratory tract consists of the lungs, which contain the bronchi, bronchioles, and alveoli.

The pharynx (the throat) is divided into three regions: the nasopharynx, which serves as a passageway for air only, and the oropharynx and the laryngopharynx, which function as a passageway for both air and food. The nasopharynx is connected to the middle ear by the auditory eustachian tubes, the obstruction of which often results in otitis media.

The larynx is also called the voice box. When an individual swallows, the epiglottis covers the entrance of the larynx to prevent food or liquid from entering the lungs. Normally, if anything other than air enters the larynx, a cough reflex is triggered that expels the substance. Because this protective reflex does not occur in an unconscious individual, aspiration is more likely to occur in such a patient.

The trachea (the windpipe) divides into the right and left primary bronchi, which further divide several times into smaller segments, the respiratory bronchioles and the terminal bronchioles. The right bronchus is shorter, wider, and straighter than the left bronchus. As a consequence, a foreign substance is more likely to enter the right bronchus, affecting the right lung.

The lungs are enveloped by the pleurae, which consist of a visceral layer and a parietal layer. Irritation of the parietal pleura will cause pain because of the sensory pain fibers in this layer. A small amount of lubricating fluid is found in between the two layers of the pleural space.

The right lung has three lobes; the left lung has two lobes. The lungs contain millions of alveoli, which collectively provide an enormous surface on which gas exchange can occur. The alveoli also produce surfactant, which reduces surface tension and facilitates alveolar expansion.

DISORDERS AND CONDITIONS

ACUTE RESPIRATORY DISTRESS SYNDROME

Acute respiratory distress syndrome (ARDS), often characterized by pulmonary edema, may result from direct or indirect insult to the lungs. Subsequently, increased membrane permeability causes fluid to accumulate in the lungs, affecting gas exchange owing to both the nonfunctional alveoli and the noncompliance (stiffening) of the lungs. Most patients with ARDS develop progressive hypoxemia (insufficient blood oxygenation) that is unresponsive to additional oxygen administration, which can in turn lead to acute respiratory failure.

Predisposing factors for developing ARDS vary widely, from fluid overload, drug overdose, smoke inhalation, gastric content aspiration, sepsis, shock, and serious trauma to pulmonary embolism.

Main Symptoms

Manifestations of ARDS may occur within hours or days of direct or indirect lung injury, including the following symptoms:

- Restlessness and decreased level of consciousness
- Dyspnea (difficulty breathing), tachypnea (increased respiration rate), and crackles (hissing sounds) auscultated over the lung fields
- Hypoxemia (with falling PaO_2 [partial pressure of oxygen] level), unresponsive to additional O_2 administration, and hypercapnia (increased serum carbon dioxide), in which O_2 is unable to cross the membrane of the alveoli as usual

If not corrected, respiratory distress may quickly become life threatening, resulting in a fatal event such as ventricular fibrillation.

Selected Nursing Tips

1. Identify at-risk patients and take preventive measures. Be alert to patients' early signs of hypoxemia, such as changes in level of consciousness and increased restlessness.
2. Treat underlying causes; prevent progression and complications of ARDS. Support ventilation with appropriate means, and reduce anxiety to decrease oxygen consumption. Monitor arterial blood gas (ABG) and lab values and prevent potential respiratory acidosis or increased $PaCO_2$ (partial pressure of carbon dioxide). Maintain blood pressure; correct fluid and electrolyte imbalances to prevent dysrhythmia.
3. Prevention and early recognition of multiple-organ dysfunction or failure are essential.

4. Proper positioning of the patient can facilitate postural draining and mobilize secretions; placing the patient in an upright position, if possible, may promote lung expansion. (Ask close-ended questions that can be answered with "yes" or "no" to reduce oxygen expenditure and difficulty breathing.)

5. Mechanical ventilation with positive end-expiratory pressure (PEEP) may help patients with ARDS avoid end-expiratory alveolar collapse and improve oxygenation in conjunction with treatment of the causative conditions. Assess the patient's oxygen saturation rate and respiratory status after placing the patient on a ventilator.

6. To minimize risks for developing ARDS, maintain patients' fluid balance to prevent fluid overload; provide adequate fluid replacement to patients experiencing hypovolemia (decreased blood volume).

Point to Consider

If a patient who has recently sustained smoke or chemical inhalation exhibits severe hypoxia (deficient oxygen supply to the tissues due to inadequate oxygenation), along with diaphoresis and dyspnea, the onset of ARDS may be suspected. Near-drowning (in which the lungs become filled with fluid) may potentially cause ARDS.

Precautions

1. Monitor the patient's vital signs and lab results closely; this condition could deteriorate quickly, and arrhythmia (irregular heart beat) may result from factors such as hypoxemia (decreased serum oxygen concentration), acidosis, and electrolyte imbalance. A variety of treatment approaches and technologies may need to be employed as ordered, including oxygen administration or mechanical ventilation.

2. A change in level of consciousness can indicate insufficient oxygen supply to the brain. Cyanosis is frequently a late sign of respiratory distress.

ASTHMA

Asthma often results from the airway becoming overresponsive or hypersensitive to various stimuli, which in turn leads to episodic bronchial spasms and constriction. This condition is recurrent and usually reversible. It is characterized with inflammation and airflow limitation. The patient with asthma may develop mucosal edema, profuse mucus production, and difficulty breathing. Episodes are often triggered by specific allergens to which the patient is sensitive (e.g., pollen, medications, food additives) or provoked by certain conditions that cause bronchial spasm (e.g., exercise in extreme temperature).

In status asthmaticus, the patient experiences a prolonged asthma attack that does not respond to initial or conventional treatment. Status asthmaticus has the potential to cause respiratory failure, which may be indicated by an absence of wheezing in a patient who has been wheezing and visibly uncomfortable with inaudible breath sounds and ineffective cough.

Main Symptoms

- Inspiratory and expiratory wheezes, often audible
- Shortness of breath, increased pulse, and perspiration
- Productive cough
- Chest tightness resulting from reduced movement of air through narrowed bronchial airways

The onset of status asthmaticus is often accompanied by confusion, diaphoresis, lethargy, and cyanosis.

Selected Nursing Tips

1. Assess patients' respiratory status and manage their symptoms; obtain a health history to identify precipitating factors, including allergens or environmental irritants. Nursing management also includes patient education and prevention of exacerbations.
2. When patients with asthma are having difficulty breathing and wheezing, the nurse may sit them up and administer

breathing treatment as ordered (often a bronchodilator) with either an inhaler or a nebulizer. Wheezing occurs as air moves through airways that have become narrowed due to bronchospasm and increased mucus production. The nurse may also administer oxygen as indicated.

3. Patients with asthma or chronic obstructive pulmonary disease (COPD) are often prescribed two metered-dose inhalers (MDIs), containing a bronchodilator and a steroid, respectively. Using a bronchodilator inhaler containing albuterol (Proventil) first may help open up the airway, thereby facilitating more effective delivery of the second (steroid) medication to the lungs. Steroid inhalation is used primarily to reduce bronchial inflammation and mucus secretions.

4. Inhaled steroids, such as beclomethasone (an anti-inflammatory immunosuppressant agent), for asthma can suppress the normal flora (beneficial organisms) in the mouth, giving rise to oral candidiasis (yeast infection). Teach and have the patient demonstrate how to use an inhaler with a spacer. Advise the patient to rinse the mouth immediately after each use to prevent dry mouth and thrush, which may appear as a cheesy white patch on the tongue or throat. Monitor the patient's respiratory status for signs of sore throat. Patients should strictly adhere to the prescribed dose schedule. When discontinuing a steroid medication, it must be tapered off as ordered.

5. Counsel patients to remove or avoid asthma triggers, which may vary for specific individuals, but often include certain foods, pollen, mold, dust, cold air, irritating odors, and smoke.

6. Follow the treatment protocol and manage status asthmaticus so as to avoid intubation. Use other treatment options to correct hypoxia and improve ventilation, including administering medications and supplemental oxygen as ordered to reduce bronchospasm and improve patients' general oxygenation.

Points to Consider

1. Albuterol (Proventil, Ventolin) and levalbuterol (Xopenex) are bronchodilators. The therapeutic effects of these adrenergic agonists include relieving bronchial muscle spasm by relaxing the smooth muscle and reducing airway resistance.

2. Ipratropium (Atrovent), an anticholinergic agent, causes bronchodilation and inhibits nasal secretion production. It is not indicated for immediate bronchospasm relief. This medication is often used together with albuterol (a bronchodilator) in the form of Combivent or DuoNeb for nebulizer-treatment use, as albuterol relieves bronchospasm. Follow the guidelines for proper inhaler use; make sure the patient does not take more than two inhalations concurrently, which can negate the broncho-dilating effect.

3. Severe asthma attack may cause respiratory acidosis with increased arterial partial pressure of carbon dioxide ($PaCO_2$), decreased partial pressure of oxygen (PaO_2), and decreased pH (acidosis) due to fatigue-induced alveolar hypoventilation.

Precaution

Cessation of wheezing breath sounds in a patient with status asthmaticus may indicate an impending respiratory obstruction. Carefully evaluate the patient with status asthmaticus to avoid misinterpreting the reduction in wheezing as an improvement of the patient's condition.

ATELECTASIS

Atelectasis, or incomplete expansion or collapse of the lung alveoli, may result from decreased breathing or reduced alveolar ventilation. Its risk factors and causes include altered breathing patterns (e.g., shallow breathing due to pain), secretion retention, immobility, increased abdominal pressure, and airway function alterations. Because gas exchange occurs in the alveolar membranes, impaired lung expansion leads to a reduction in the surface area available for gas exchange, subsequently causing hypoxia.

Main Symptoms

- Dyspnea to different degrees depending on the underlying cause, the extent of compromised condition, and the severity of hypoxia
- Diminished or absent lung sounds on the affected areas
- Anxiety
- Tachycardia and cyanosis

Selected Nursing Tips

1. Identify the risk factors in patients with compromised respiratory status and take steps to improve breathing effectiveness.
2. A simple and effective way to optimize patients' respiration and prevent atelectasis is to have them breathe deeply and cough at times to maintain an open airway. If coughing causes pain at an incision site, teach the postoperative patient to splint the incision with a pillow before coughing. Patients tend to cooperate when pain is alleviated with adequate analgesics.
3. Frequent repositioning and assisting early ambulation may help prevent atelectasis in at-risk patients. Elevating the head and chest properly may promote airway clearance and lung expansion.
4. Using incentive (spirometry) breathing may help patients with certain acute conditions, such as after surgery or having a fractured rib, to breathe deeply on a regular basis to prevent pulmonary complications. Ambulating is encouraged but cannot be done as conveniently and frequently as using the spirometry.
5. Encourage fluid intake, as appropriate, and humidify the inhaled air to loosen and mobilize secretions.

Points to Consider

1. Deep breathing allows the diaphragm to descend, expanding the ventilating surface and thereby reducing the patient's risk of developing atelectasis.

2. Chest percussion, postural drainage, and incentive spirometry may be utilized in addition to medication, if prescribed. Suction as needed, especially if the patient is intubated. Auscultate lung sounds to determine if suction is needed; obtain the patient's vital signs, and provide oxygenation before the procedure.

3. Severe or massive atelectasis may result in acute respiratory distress, especially in patients with coexisting pulmonary diseases. Other respiratory-care measures may be employed by practitioners as indicated for severe cases, including endotracheal intubation and mechanical ventilation. The underlying causes of atelectasis must always be addressed or removed.

4. For most patients, a pulse oximetry reading provides information about the percentage of oxygenated (oxygen-carrying) hemoglobin. For instance, an arterial O_2 saturation level of 97% usually indicates that 97% of the total hemoglobin attachments for O_2 are oxygen saturated. However, the readings are less accurate with O_2 saturations below 75% and unreliable with poor peripheral perfusion.

Precautions

1. Sedatives will depress breathing and the cough reflex; they should be administered with discretion per the physician's orders.

2. Be vigilant for signs of severe atelectasis, such as dyspnea or hypoxia. These conditions may be indicated by low O_2 saturation rate, which can be easily monitored via pulse oximetry.

CHRONIC OBSTRUCTIVE PULMONARY DISEASE

Chronic obstructive pulmonary disease (COPD) usually includes a chronic inflammation (abnormal inflammatory response) component as well as progressive airflow limitation.

The classification of diseases subsumed under the COPD heading has been changing over the years as results emerge from ongoing research. Discussed in this section (extremely briefly) are chronic bronchitis and emphysema.

Even though COPD cannot be fully reversed, it is treatable. In fact, this condition is often preventable, as it is frequently related to exposure to smoke or environmental pollutants. It is common for bronchitis, emphysema, and asthma to coexist in patients with COPD, with their symptoms overlapping.

Main Symptoms

Clinical features of chronic bronchitis may include the following symptoms:

- Productive cough, excessive mucus secretion, decreased airway clearance due to airway inflammation, and increased susceptibility to respiratory infection
- Activity intolerance and exertional dyspnea
- Edema, weight gain, and cyanosis

In patients with emphysema, impaired gas exchange often results from damage to the alveolar walls, which causes decreased elastic recoil and reduces the surface area available for gas exchange. Exhalation may become difficult, resulting in air trapping and hypoxia. Manifestations of these developments may include the following signs and symptoms:

- Dyspnea and barrel chest
- Anorexia, thin appearance, and malaise
- Having a sense of air hunger, using accessory muscles to breathe through pursed lips, and often assuming a tripod position—that is, sitting with arms supported on a table

In later stages, hypoxemia may be further worsened, and hypercapnia and respiratory acidosis may occur. Peripheral edema and pulmonary congestion may indicate the cardiac involvement.

Patients with advanced COPD (especially emphysema) are typically barrel-chested (with hyper-inflated chest and flattened diaphragm on chest X-ray) owing to the incomplete CO_2 elimination associated with this condition. The neck muscles may be overly developed and the neck veins distended.

Both chronic bronchitis and emphysema may have some characteristics in common:

- Possible productive cough
- Dyspnea on exertion, progressing to dyspnea at rest
- Diminished breath sounds, use of accessory muscles to breathe, and airflow limitations

Selected Nursing Tips

1. Provide low-dose oxygen as needed. It is very important that patients with COPD not receive high-dose oxygen, as this treatment may reduce or stop their own drive to breathe, necessitating the use of an Ambu (resuscitation) bag to ventilate the patient. (Note that there are other theories regarding the underlying causes of this condition.)

2. Encourage patients with chronic bronchitis to increase their fluid intake, if not contraindicated. Ensuring adequate hydration may help mobilize secretions for expectoration and replace fluid loss from pathologies such as fever or other causes.

3. Teach patients to employ diaphragmatic/abdominal breathing, which relieves the accessory muscles of much of the work of respiration and improves ventilation.

4. Coarse crackles, rhonchi (snoring sound heard during auscultation), and wheezes are abnormal lung sounds associated with exacerbations of COPD. They often occur

secondary to respiratory infection, as air passes through a secretion-obstructed narrowing airway.

5. If a patient with COPD becomes restless due to dyspnea, initial nursing actions usually include starting low-dose oxygen administration and assisting the patient to sit up, if possible, to facilitate breathing. Monitor the patient's oxygenation status with a pulse oximeter.

6. Patients with COPD are highly recommended to obtain the influenza and pneumococcal vaccinations, per protocol, as preventive measures. The accumulation of respiratory secretions due to ineffective airway clearance in these patients is the main risk factor for pulmonary infection.

7. Encourage patients to adopt healthy habits and participate in regular aerobic exercise, which promotes cardiac fitness and increases activity tolerance. Teach patients how to recognize the symptoms of respiratory infection and potential complications of COPD.

Points to Consider

1. Persuade patients to stop smoking, even though it is a hard habit to break. If smoking cessation is successful, it will be a cost-effective way to prevent the development or halt the progression of COPD. Use of tobacco can affect the airway-cleansing mechanism and increase mucus accumulation, causing more irritation to the lungs. In addition, one of the by-products of smoking is carbon monoxide, which renders hemoglobin incapable of carrying oxygen. (Carbon monoxide from cigarette smoking can saturate the body's hemoglobin, which makes pulse oximetry O_2 saturation values inaccurate in patients who are smokers.) Secondhand smoke can also contribute to the development of COPD.

2. Some over-the-counter medications may thicken bronchial secretions, like antihistamines such as diphenhydramine (Benadryl). Patients with COPD should use these medications with caution.

3. Pursed-lip breathing (or whistling while exhaling) is a beneficial form of exercise for patients with COPD, as it promotes relaxation and keeps the bronchi open, allowing more effective exhalation of the carbon dioxide trapped in the alveoli.

4. Rust-colored sputum from a patient with COPD may indicate blood in the sputum and require further assessment to rule out pneumonia or other complications.

5. Right-sided heart failure may result from COPD because of the development of pulmonary hypertension. Typical signs to be monitored include peripheral edema and jugular vein distension, among others.

6. Polycythemia (excessive production of red blood cells) may occur secondary to COPD as a result of the body's compensatory response to chronic hypoxia; higher-than-normal blood viscosity increases risk of thrombosis.

Precaution

Oxygen administered at a rate exceeding 2–3 L/m may depress or eliminate the hypoxic respiratory drive in patients with COPD. One theory explains this effect by proposing that the breathing drive in patients with COPD is linked to a low blood O_2 level (hypoxia), whereas a high CO_2 level stimulates the respiratory center in the medulla of people with healthy lungs to breathe.

COR PULMONALE

In cor pulmonale, the right ventricle of the heart is enlarged (hypertrophic). This condition often emerges secondary to pulmonary disorders affecting the right side of the heart, such as COPD with pulmonary hypertension, resulting in right-sided heart failure. Lung disorders that cause hypoxemia, resulting in pulmonary blood-vessel constriction and vascular-bed reduction, may potentially lead to cor pulmonale. Cor pulmonale often occurs late in the course of irreversible lung diseases with a poor prognosis.

Main Symptoms

Patients with cor pulmonale may or may not exhibit signs of heart failure when the heart can compensate for the increased pulmonary vascular resistance. Clinical manifestations often reflect underlying disorder, and consist of mostly respiratory symptoms:

- Chronic productive cough
- Exertional dyspnea and wheezing
- Fatigue and weakness

When right-sided heart failure develops in cor pulmonale, patients may present with the following symptoms:

- Resting dyspnea, tachypnea, and orthopnea (labored breathing while lying flat)
- Weight gain, dependent edema, distended neck veins, and signs of right-sided heart failure
- A weak pulse, reflecting decreased cardiac output

Selected Nursing Tips

1. Manage cor pulmonale by reducing hypoxemia, increasing activity tolerance, and treating pulmonary problems that would induce heart failure.
2. Provide small and frequent meals, as patients with cor pulmonale tire easily. Fluid and salt restriction, if so ordered, may reduce fluid retention.
3. Provide oxygen therapy and teach pursed-lip breathing; suggest bed rest to decrease oxygen demand as indicated.
4. If the patient is receiving diuretics, such as potassium-depleting furosemide (Lasix) and potassium-sparing spironolactone (Aldactone), monitor serum electrolytes closely, especially potassium levels. Either hyperkalemia or hypokalemia can cause a dangerous cardiac arrhythmia.
5. Emphasize the importance of adhering to the treatment regimen.

Point to Consider

Provide teaching about the need for lifestyle modifications, including adequate rest, weighing oneself daily, and reporting signs of edema, weight gain, or respiratory infection such as an increased amount of sputum, fever, or wheezing.

Precaution

Monitor the patient's oxygenation status and arterial blood gas levels. Watch for signs of respiratory failure, such as restlessness, confusion, low oxygen saturation rate, and labored breathing.

CYSTIC FIBROSIS

Cystic fibrosis (CF), a genetic disorder, is characterized by dysfunction of the exocrine glands, which causes secretions to be thick and sweat high in salt content. The functions of multiple organs can be affected, including the lungs, sweat glands, intestines, liver, and pancreas. Patients may develop bronchial mucus plugging, inflammation, and potentially bronchiectasis, progressively losing lung function. Cysts may occur in the lungs, and some portion of the glands may become fibrotic and scarred.

Main Symptoms

- Profuse thick, sticky respiratory secretions; impaired airway clearance; and inflammation
- Fibrotic/pathologic changes in the pancreas, resulting in reduced pancreatic enzymes and malabsorption of fat and protein, leading to other gastrointestinal (GI) problems
- Steatorrhea (bulky fatty stools) because of undigested fats
- Salty sweat (containing increased sodium and chloride) due to sweat gland dysfunction, potentially causing hyponatremia and hypochloremia

Patients with CF are often malnourished. In addition, they are predisposed to electrolyte imbalances and respiratory complications.

Selected Nursing Tips

1. Support the patient and family throughout the disease process in an interdisciplinary therapy approach; address end-of-life concerns as warranted.

2. Encourage consumption of a diet low in fat, but high in protein and calories. Provide necessary supplementation of fat-soluble vitamins (A, D, E, and K) and added salt as prescribed or recommended.

3. Educate patients that taking pancreatic enzymes as ordered (with a generous amount of liquid) can aid the absorption of the nutrients in the meals and snacks ingested.

4. Arrange for prescribed chest physiotherapy, such as postural drainage, chest percussion, vibration (or vibrating vests treatment), and breathing exercises to promote removal of secretions from the lungs.

5. Increasing fluid intake, as appropriate, can help dilute secretions and facilitate expectoration. Monitor for signs of complications and prevent respiratory infection.

Point to Consider

Recommend the use of humidifiers to decrease the patient's susceptibility to respiratory infection, as appropriate.
Teach proper maintenance of the humidifier to prevent its contamination.

Precaution

Antihistamines have a drying effect, which can make airway clearance more difficult. Patients with CF should, in general, avoid the use of these medications.

INFLUENZA

Influenza, or the flu, refers to an acute viral respiratory infection, with type A and B influenza viruses being more common. Influenza is highly contagious when symptoms are present in patients. The pathogen can be spread by droplets or through contact with contaminated items handled by the patient.

Excellent hand hygiene is an important step to prevent the spread of the virus.

Main Symptoms

The onset is often abrupt. In mild cases, symptoms may resemble those of the common cold:

- Fever, chills, headache, malaise, and myalgia (muscle pain)
- Profuse nasal drainage
- Sore throat and cough

Selected Nursing Tips

1. For uncomplicated influenza, treatment consists of establishing an accurate diagnosis, symptomatic relief, and complication prevention.
2. Thorough hand washing is an essential part of universal precautions.
3. Antibiotics are not effective in treating viral infections, including viral influenza, unless they are complicated by bacterial infection.
4. Advise patients to avoid crowds to protect themselves from bacterial infection as well as to contain the spread of the virus. Increase fluid intake and ensure adequate rest. Watch for signs of secondary pneumonia, such as auscultated crackles or purulent sputum.
5. Educate patients per protocol about vaccination, including its possible adverse effects and its contraindications in certain populations.
6. Aspirin may reduce fever and pain, in addition to having anti-inflammatory and anticoagulant effects. This medication is contraindicated for children due to its possible association with an acute febrile illness (Reye's syndrome).

Point to Consider

Influenza viruses have a remarkable ability to mutate over time, which necessitates the need for annual vaccination against new strains. Some of the evolving strains may have pandemic potential, as they constantly change. Take preventive measures as required by public health authorities.

Precaution

Patients who are allergic to eggs, feathers, chickens, or who have histories of certain conditions or disorders, such as Guillain–Barré syndrome, should consult the practitioner regarding flu prevention. Alternative approaches may be adopted. However, antiviral agents such as oseltamivir (Tamiflu) or amantadine (Symmetrel) are not the same as vaccinations.

LARYNGEAL CANCER

Laryngeal cancer refers to uncontrollable malignant cell growth involving the vocal cords or some other part of the larynx. Squamous cell carcinoma is a common type. Risk factors for this disease include smoking, excessive alcohol intake, vocal abuse, and chronic laryngitis.

Main Symptoms

Manifestations may vary depending on the location of the tumor, but often include the following symptoms:

- Persistent hoarseness and cough
- Sore throat, or a feeling of a lump with burning sensation in the throat, especially when drinking hot or citrus fluids
- Dysphagia (difficulty swallowing), ulceration, and foul breath
- Dyspnea, enlarged cervical lymph nodes, and weight loss

Selected Nursing Tips

1. Before a laryngectomy, the patient's reading and writing abilities need to be assessed, and a means of communication established (e.g., the call light or a writing pad). Encourage patients to express their feelings related to fears or depression; listening can be therapeutic. Clarify any

misconceptions they may have to allay their anxiety and help them cope with the disease process, as it may pose threats to their body image and self-esteem.

2. In total laryngectomy, the patient's laryngeal structures are removed, and the tracheostomy is permanent. Precautions must be taken to prevent water from entering the stoma (e.g., no participation in water sports after the surgery). Educate the patient or caregivers to cover the stoma when showering or bathing; teach and have them demonstrate competence in performing stoma-related care.

3. Postoperatively, maintain a patent (open) airway, and clear secretions by suctioning as indicated. (The secretions are likely to increase due to the resultant structural and functional changes.) Properly raise the head of the bed to promote lymphatic drainage and decrease pressure on the suture line. Take measures to prevent aspiration pneumonia, because patients who have had laryngectomy may experience a depressed cough reflex.

4. Shortly after a patient undergoes a total laryngectomy, the nurse should closely monitor the patient for signs of dyspnea and bleeding and position the patient properly as recommended.

5. After a total laryngectomy, the patient may use alternative communication methods. For example, the patient may be taught by a speech therapist over time to learn to use "esophageal speech," in which swallowed or compressed air is expelled across constricted tissue in a controlled "belch" to create sounds and form words. Some patients may not be successful in learning this technique.

6. Patient teaching concerning self-care changes (due to the loss of functional abilities, such as sense of smell) is an important part of the nursing role. A humidifier or house plants in the home, if appropriate, may help compensate for the loss of the humidifying mechanism of the nose and pharynx until the body has adjusted to the changes.

Points to Consider

1. Prolonged use of tobacco (smoking or smokeless) and alcohol increases the risk for developing laryngeal cancer. Other risk factors include vocal straining and exposure to toxins or radiation.
2. Radiation of the head and neck after laryngectomy frequently causes xerostomia (dry mouth), stomatitis (irritation of the oral mucous membranes), and dysgeusia (reduced sense of taste).

Precautions

1. The outer tracheostomy tube should not be removed unnecessarily, because the stoma may close.
2. When moving the patient postoperatively, make sure to support the neck and head.
3. Before the postoperative patient is cleared for oral intake, the speech therapist and the radiologist may conduct a swallow study to evaluate aspiration risks.

LARYNGITIS

Laryngitis—an acute or chronic inflammation of the larynx, which contains the vocal cords—can be caused by viral or bacterial pathogens, as in an upper respiratory infection, or induced by other factors, including voice overuse, exposure to chemicals and irritants, or gastroesophageal reflux. It can also be brought on by conditions such as temperature fluctuations, nutritional deficiencies, or an immunosuppressed state.

Main Symptoms

- Mild to complete loss of voice, accompanied by red and sore throat
- Flu-like symptoms
- Possible dry cough and fever
- Pain associated with swallowing and speaking

A persistent hoarseness is often the only clinical feature of chronic laryngitis.

Selected Nursing Tips

1. Encourage patients to rest their voice and avoid smoking and/or alcohol. Anticipate their needs, and use alternative communication methods, such as a writing pad or sign language.
2. Analgesics and throat lozenges are often used to relieve the symptoms of viral infection; antibiotics are commonly prescribed for bacterial infection.
3. Underlying causes should be identified and corrected or removed. Increase fluid intake, if not contraindicated.

Points to Consider

1. Maintain humidification by taking throat lozenges, using a vaporizer in winter, and minimizing air-conditioning use in summer.
2. Laryngeal edema in severe cases may result in airway obstruction, necessitating tracheotomy preparation.

Precaution

Advise the patient to report difficulty swallowing, pinkish sputum (possible hemoptysis), or noisy breathing. Prolonged hoarseness needs to be evaluated to rule out malignancy.

LEGIONNAIRES' DISEASE

Legionnaires' disease is often characterized by multiple-system involvement in addition to respiratory infection (pneumonia). The causative bacterium, *Legionella pneumophila*, is typically transmitted via inhalation of vapors or aerosolized water droplets from a water source, especially contaminated standing warm water. Spread of the pathogen may be linked to plumbing, cooling systems, or respiratory equipment. The bacteria can also be found in soil.

Main Symptoms

- Fever, malaise, and headache
- Dyspnea and cough that eventually becomes productive
- Weakness and myalgia (muscle pains)
- Gastrointestinal problems, including diarrhea

Legionnaires' disease may also result in serious complications, including hypotension or organ failure.

Selected Nursing Tips

1. Provide circulatory and ventilation support; administer prescribed medications, such as antibiotic or antipyretic (temperature-lowering) agents.
2. Monitor the patient's status closely; replace fluids and electrolytes as ordered.
3. Encourage coughing and deep breathing to improve lung function. Watch for signs of hypoxemia, such as confusion or restlessness, which may require repositioning, suctioning, or further oxygenation therapy.
4. Advocate about proper treatment and maintenance of water systems, including any water sources for drinking, bathing, cooling, or decoration. Use prescribed (sterile) water for aerosolizing breathing treatment and clean the equipment as required to prevent contamination.

Point to Consider

Smokers and people who are immunocompromised or have chronic debilitating diseases are relatively more susceptible to Legionnaires' disease (which usually is not spread from person to person).

Precaution

Monitor patients for signs of complications, including shock (as evidenced by hypotension, thread pulse, and sweating with clammy skin) and organ failure.

LUNG CANCER

The prognosis for patients with lung cancer, a malignant tumor within the lung, varies depending on the stage at diagnosis and the growth rate of the specific cell type (e.g., small cell lung cancer versus non-small cell lung cancer and its various subtypes). Risk factors include, but are not limited to, tobacco use, secondhand smoke, exposure to harmful substances, and other predisposing conditions (e.g., lung diseases).

Main Symptoms

Lung cancer is often asymptomatic in its early stages. Eventually symptoms occur depending on many factors, such as the tumor size and location and its metastatic effects. General warning signs and possible symptoms include the following:

- A persistent cough or a change in the character of cough
- Dyspnea, wheezing, and hoarseness
- Chest pain aggravated by a deep breath
- Recurrent respiratory infections or pleural effusion
- Blood-tinged sputum (hemoptysis)
- Palpable lymph nodes
- Anorexia, weakness, and weight loss

Selected Nursing Tips

1. Assess patients' risk factors and advise them to seek additional medical attention as appropriate, because early detection and treatment are likely to increase patient survival rates.
2. Presurgery teaching should cover possible postoperative procedures, such as placement of a chest tube, IV catheter insertion, and urinary catheterization.
3. Position the postoperative patient on the recommended side that will promote drainage and lung expansion.
4. Remind the patient with terminal lung cancer experiencing severe pain to ask for analgesic medication before the pain becomes extreme.

5. Provide supportive care and teaching to minimize complications and facilitate recovery from surgery, radiation, chemotherapy, and other treatment therapies.
6. Following a one-sided pneumonectomy (removal of an entire lung), assess the trachea per protocol, as it may deviate from midline. A semi-Fowler's (30–45 degrees) position may facilitate the patient's breathing without inducing devastating fatigue.

Points to Consider

1. Proper positioning and deep breathing can reduce the patient's risk of developing complications, such as atelectasis. During inspiration, the diaphragm descends, which increases thoracic volume and lowers pressure, allowing air to rush into the alveoli.
2. Radiation may be used preoperatively to reduce tumor size for surgical excision or postoperatively as an additional therapy.

Precaution

Warn patients receiving radiation therapy against wearing restrictive clothing and being exposed to the sun. Take other protective measures as well to minimize skin breakdown.

OBSTRUCTIVE SLEEP APNEA

People who suffer from obstructive sleep apnea (OSA) characteristically experience repeated temporary cessations of breathing (apnea) during sleep. In susceptible patients, such as those who are obese or who have a large neck size, a partial or complete upper airway obstruction may occur when pharyngeal muscle tone is reduced during sleep, impeding airflow; in such individuals, the pharynx can be compressed during inspiration by surrounding soft tissues. Recurrent apneic episodes may decrease blood O_2 saturation and increase carbon dioxide concentration.

Main Symptoms

- Loud snoring and frequent awakening at night to make breathing possible
- Insomnia
- Daytime sleepiness at inappropriate times
- Morning headaches due to hypercapnia, which may cause cerebral vasodilation (and headache)
- Inability to concentrate and impaired memory
- Personality changes, irritability, and typically lack of awareness of the sleep apnea problem

Selected Nursing Tips

1. Make appropriate referrals, as many individuals may not realize the seriousness of this condition and go undiagnosed. Assist patients to further identify the causes and related problems.
2. Instruct patients to minimize their use of alcohol or sedatives. Explain to the susceptible individuals the risk factors associated with OSA, such as obesity and altered upper airway structures; encourage weight reduction when indicated.
3. Anticipate patients' knowledge deficits regarding treatment options or possible complications, and provide education to enhance their understanding to facilitate their compliance with the mask use for continuous positive airway pressure (CPAP) or bilevel positive airway pressure (BiPAP) while sleeping.

Points to Consider

1. Continuous positive airway pressure is primarily used by patients with OSA who can breathe independently; it is intended to prevent the hypoxemia that may occur during sleep. The machine blows enough air into the patient's nose (and/or mouth) to maintain a level of positive airway pressure that keeps the alveoli open for the entire breathing cycle. Some patients cannot adapt to exhaling against the

high pressure delivered by CPAP; in such cases, bilevel positive airway pressure therapy may be a better choice.

2. The use of BiPAP can provide cooperative patients who can breathe spontaneously with needed support of both higher inspiratory and lower expiratory positive airway pressure in conjunction with oxygen.

3. Assessing the patient's oxygen saturation at night with pulse oximetry may provide useful information for evaluating the patient's oxygenation and the need for further treatment.

4. A variety of treatment approaches are possible. Surgical management of OSA is reserved for patients whose symptoms cannot be relieved with other measures. Benefits need to be weighed against the adverse effects of the treatments, including medications.

Precaution

Obstructive sleep apnea may induce hypertension and other abnormalities. When recurrent apneic episodes result in hypercapnia and hypoxia, the subsequent sympathetic response poses an increased risk for developing serious cardiovascular problems, including pulmonary hypertension.

PNEUMONIA

In pneumonia, there is inflammation of the lungs due to infectious organisms or other conditions and offending agents (as in pneumonitis, which predisposes the patient to infection), consequently diminishing the optimal gas exchange. Numerous factors may increase a patient's risk of developing pneumonia, including aspirated food, inhaled gases, contaminated breathing treatment equipment, prolonged immobility, smoking, alcohol intoxication, and impaired breathing or airway clearance. Various terms may be used to describe pneumonia based on different criteria or etiologies, such as "hospital-acquired pneumonia" and "aspiration pneumonia," among others.

Main Symptoms

Manifestations depend on the type of pneumonia, the etiologic agents, and coexisting underlying conditions. Presentations of bacterial pneumonia are possibly associated with the following symptoms:

- Diminished breath sounds upon auscultation over a consolidated, fluid-filled area, and crackles
- Productive coughing with greenish sputum and positive sputum culture
- Pleuritic chest pain worsened by deep breathing or cough
- Fever, chills, tachypnea, tachycardia, and malaise
- Chest X-ray showing areas of consolidation (solidification) or patchy infiltrates

Older patients with COPD who also develop pneumonia may not exhibit the typical signs. Instead, they may simply appear lethargic, confused, or dehydrated, with changes in respiratory status.

Selected Nursing Tips

1. Obtain a sputum sample for a culture and sensitivity test before antibiotic therapy is initiated. The sputum specimen is optimally collected in the early morning from a deep cough after brushing the teeth.
2. During the acute phase of pneumonia, maintaining bed rest may minimize the body's metabolic demand for oxygen.
3. Monitor lab results and maintain fluid and electrolyte balance; provide adequate nutrition. During and after eating, the patient's head and chest should be properly elevated to reduce the risk of aspiration pneumonia.
4. Patients of advanced age and those with long-term illness or in group-living settings are more susceptible to pneumonia. Annual influenza vaccination is usually encouraged and vaccination against pneumococcal and influenza

infections is recommended, per protocol, for high-risk patients, such as those with chronic heart or lung disease.

5. Encourage immobile or postoperative patients to cough, turn, and deep breathe. To reduce pain while coughing, the patient may splint his or her chest with a pillow.

Point to Consider

Severe acute respiratory syndrome (SARS) refers to a viral respiratory infection, which is highly contagious. It is mainly transmitted via the respiratory tract by means of airborne droplets or contact with droplet-contaminated objects. Patients with SARS initially may experience fever, headache, and general discomfort. Cough and difficulty breathing may develop later. Currently, management of patients with SARS is primarily supportive; the efficacy of antiviral therapy is unclear so far.

Precaution

To prevent tube-feeding–related aspiration pneumonia, check the placement of the feeding tube and the residual per protocol before administering enteral feeding to patients. Keep the patient's chest and head properly elevated during and after the feeding.

PNEUMOTHORAX

To maintain lung inflation, the pressure inside the double-layered pleurae normally is lower than the atmospheric pressure (negative pressure). In pneumothorax, the negative pressure in the pleurae is disrupted due to the presence of air, which causes the affected lung or portion of lung to collapse.

Causative factors may range from chest injury to spontaneous air bleb rupture, causing air to enter the pleural space. When a partial or complete lung collapse occurs, gaseous exchange and cardiac output will be impaired. Pneumothorax is considered an emergency and requires immediate medical intervention.

Main Symptoms

The manifestations of pneumothorax are related to the size of the affected area and the underlying conditions or causes, with specific terms being used to describe the variants.

In a *spontaneous* (or simple) pneumothorax, the patient may not have sustained trauma. This type of pneumothorax can occur in a healthy person through an air bleb rupture, producing no obvious symptoms. It may also be associated with certain lung diseases, such as severe emphysema.

In a *traumatic* pneumothorax (after having sustained major injury to the chest), circulatory function may be seriously affected. When both air and blood are found in the chest cavity, the condition may be termed a *hemopneumothorax.*

In *tension* pneumothorax, the air taken in with each breath increases pressure (tension) in the pleural space, but it cannot escape or be expelled. This condition may potentially cause the lung to collapse and lead to mediastinal shift, in which the heart, great vessels, and trachea shift to the unaffected side.

In general, patients with pneumothorax may display the following respiratory symptoms:

- Sudden, sharp pleural chest pain worsened by breathing, along with shortness of breath
- Decreased breath sounds on the affected side
- Asymmetrical chest movement with signs of shortness of breath
- Cyanosis, diaphoresis, and tachycardia
- Anxiety and air hunger

Selected Nursing Tips

1. Emergency care and interventions are required to treat pneumothorax that affects circulatory function, including tension pneumothorax and traumatic pneumothorax. Conservative treatment may include monitoring of vital signs, bed rest, and oxygen therapy.

2. Negative pressure in the pleural space may need to be re-established with medical interventions by or under the guidance of medical experts. Monitor the patient's oxygen saturation rate and vital signs; ensure adequate oxygenation. Observe the patient closely and report promptly any signs of complications, such as pressure in the chest, significant changes in vital signs, difficulty breathing, hemorrhage, or cyanosis.

3. In a trauma patient, diminished or absent breath sounds over the affected areas with sudden sharp chest pain related to breathing and dyspnea should arouse suspicion for pneumothorax with impaired lung function. Immediate proper actions and interventions are indicated.

4. In hemothorax, blood is present in the pleural space, often resulting from chest injury. When the excessive blood is removed with a chest tube, it may be reinfused within hours as per protocol. The blood for autotransfusion must be collected and filtered to eliminate air and other substances; a special autotransfusion machine may be used for that purpose.

5. Oxygen saturation can be monitored continuously using pulse oximetry; providing optimal oxygenation is essential in case of pneumothorax.

Points to Consider

1. Managing chest tube drainage per guidelines and orders is an important aspect of nursing care. The chest tube is used to remove air and excess fluid from the pleurae, thereby allowing the affected lung to re-expand. As with any invasive procedure, before a chest tube is inserted in an alert and oriented patient, the patient or his or her guardian must sign an informed consent form.

2. The traditional water seal chest drainage system has been largely replaced with newer technology (e.g., dry-suction water-seal drainage or dry-suction one-way valve system). The nurse should be familiar with the safety mechanisms of the system being used.

3. Make sure that the drainage tubing does not kink, loop, or interfere with drainage function or the patient's movement. Secure all the connections; air leaking or trapping in the pleural space can lead to tension pneumothorax. Correct the causes of leakage, as evidenced by constant bubbling in the water-seal chamber in a wet system (or as detected by the air-leak indicator in a dry system with a one-way valve), and report a not-correctable leakage, obstruction, or other problems to the physician. Normally, the water in the water-seal chamber (in wet systems) fluctuates with the patient's breathing, reflecting the pressure in the pleurae, with intermittent gentle bubbles being noted (before the lung is fully re-expanded).

4. The drainage system must be kept below the level of the patient's chest. The tubing should not be clamped to prevent tension pneumothorax, except momentarily when absolutely necessary or specifically ordered.

5. Position patients in good body alignment, and reposition them at proper intervals. Deep breathing or coughing promotes drainage and removal of secretions and helps prevent atelectasis.

6. To prevent atelectasis, analgesics may be needed if a patient with a chest tube experiences severe pain when taking deep breaths.

Precaution

Pneumothorax is a life-threatening disorder, which may produce signs of severe respiratory distress, especially in case of tension pneumothorax, and which requires immediate medical intervention.

PULMONARY EDEMA

In pulmonary edema, abnormal fluid buildup occurs in the alveoli and interstitial spaces of the lungs, often secondary to a cardiac disorder (e.g., myocardial infarction or an exacerbation of chronic heart failure) or a non-cardiac disorder that causes fluid retention (e.g., renal failure). This fluid buildup results in decreased lung compliance and gas exchange.

A wide range of conditions can predispose the patients to pulmonary edema, including excessive volume of intravenous (IV) fluid, hypervolemia, acute respiratory distress syndrome, trauma, severe burns, shock, and severe nutritional deficiency (hypoalbuminemia with decreased colloid osmotic pressure). Pulmonary edema, a life-threatening medical emergency, can develop either gradually or rapidly (in a few minutes).

Main Symptoms

- Restlessness (resulting from inadequate blood flow to the brain), anxiety, and confusion
- Difficulty breathing and air hunger, especially upon exertion or while lying down
- Blood-tinged, pink, frothy sputum
- Signs of hypoxia (e.g., cool, cyanotic, clammy skin)
- Signs of pulmonary congestion, such as a sense of "drowning" or "suffocating" in one's own secretions
- Arterial blood gas analysis and pulse oximetry indicating worsening hypoxemia (or other abnormalities)

Selected Nursing Tips

1. Monitor susceptible patients for early signs of pulmonary edema, especially breathing problems, abnormal breath sounds, tachycardia, and signs of pulmonary congestion, such as auscultated crackles or peripheral edema, which may possibly indicate pulmonary fluid accumulation.
2. Pulmonary edema is a life-threatening emergency. When signs of acute pulmonary edema are noted, immediate nursing actions are required. Stay with the patient and call for help. Notify the practitioner promptly. Initiate other interventions per protocol and as appropriate, such as oxygen supplementation, cardiac monitoring, starting an IV line, and suctioning the patient as indicated, in collaboration with the healthcare team to correct fluid overload, improve

cardiac functioning, and promote pulmonary gas exchange. (In severe cases, endotracheal intubation and mechanical ventilation may be required for some patients.)

3. To reduce the heart's workload, the patient needs to use stress- and activity-reducing techniques, such as using a bedside commode. Raise the head of the bed, as appropriate. Placing the patient's legs in a dependent position at times may decrease venous return and pulmonary congestion.

4. Monitor lab values, fluid intake, and urine output. Instruct the patient to keep a daily weight record at home to assess fluid status. Identify and avoid precipitating factors; control fluid and salt intake to prevent fluid retention and the recurrence of pulmonary edema.

Point to Consider

A potassium supplement may be ordered for patients who take potassium-depleting diuretics, such as furosemide (Lasix); monitor their serum potassium level. When patients are on potassium-sparing diuretics, such as spironolactone (Aldactone), they should avoid consumption of potassium-containing salt substitutes.

Precaution

Narcotics are not commonly used in patients with respiratory distress. However, morphine may be prescribed for dyspnea from pulmonary edema that is unrelated to chemical respiratory irritants. Monitor for its side effects, especially respiratory depression. Ventilation support should be readily available.

PULMONARY EMBOLISM

In pulmonary embolism (PE), there is a blockage in the pulmonary arterial bed, which impedes pulmonary blood flow. It may be caused by a dislodged thrombus (blood clot) or another type of embolus (of a solid, liquid, or gaseous mass), such as tumor cells, bone marrow, amniotic fluid, or air. PE frequently results from thrombi that originate in the deep veins, commonly in the calf or thigh.

As a result of PE, pulmonary vascular resistance may increase. Gas exchange will be severely impaired with potentially fatal consequences, if this acute condition is not recognized and treated promptly.

Main Symptoms

The manifestations of PE can be nonspecific. The clinical picture may vary with the location and the severity of the occlusion, or may mimic that of other cardiopulmonary disorders. Patients may develop the following symptoms:

- Shortness of breath and rapid, weak pulse
- Sudden chest pain that is associated with breathing
- Cough with blood-tinged sputum from alveolar damage
- Apprehension due to sudden reduction in oxygenation
- Fever
- Diaphoresis, syncope (fainting)

These symptoms can develop rapidly. Early detection is essential: Failure to recognize this condition early and delay in treatment are often the cause of PE-related death.

Selected Nursing Tips

1. Pulmonary embolism is a life-threatening emergency requiring immediate medical intervention to stabilize the patient's cardiac and pulmonary systems as per protocol.
2. Identifying vulnerable patients and taking measures to prevent clot formation are important roles for nurses. Advise patients on ways to prevent thrombosis, such as engaging in safe, moderate exercise and avoiding prolonged immobility or restrictive clothing.
3. Patients on bed rest who are at risk for thrombosis should avoid pressure on the popliteal area. For example, they should not place a pillow under their knees, as it may impede the circulation and promote clot formation.

4. To prevent venous stasis and reduce the risks for PE, encourage patients to walk as soon as appropriate after surgery or when the condition is stabilized.

5. Administer medication and oxygen as prescribed; maintain cardiopulmonary function during the treatment of emboli. Carefully monitor patients' thrombolytic or anticoagulant therapy and lab test results.

6. Emphasize the importance of compliance with possibly long-term therapy to prevent the recurrence of PE. Check patients' medication lists to report concurrent use of aspirin or other nonsteroidal anti-inflammatory drugs while they are on anticoagulants to prevent bleeding.

7. When patients with PE are discharged from the hospital, provide education on preventing dehydration by taking extra fluids to thin the blood when necessary (e.g., on a long trip).

Points to Consider

1. Heparin and warfarin (Coumadin) may inhibit the growth of existing clots and reduce the likelihood that new clots will form. Their dosage is usually adjusted frequently based on the results of blood coagulation studies, such as the international normalized ratio (INR), per protocol. It is necessary to cross-check the dosage with a coworker to ensure dosage accuracy. Patients should also be closely monitored for signs of bleeding. Advise patients to take measures to prevent tissue injuries (e.g., using a safety shaving razor or soft toothbrush). There are a number of anticoagulant agents, including enoxaparin (Lovenox); when an anticoagulant is used, monitor the patient for signs of bleeding (or anemia), among other side effects.

2. Patients with acute massive pulmonary embolism may need thrombolytic therapy, using agents such as alteplase (Activase), a tissue plasminogen activator. These agents should be given within the first 3 hours of the onset of the

symptoms or within the time frame directed per protocol. Closely observe the medication's administration guidelines. Maintain continuous cardiac monitoring on patients receiving thrombolytic therapy for signs of arrhythmia; assess for signs of overt bleeding or having occult blood in any body substance.

3. Leaving an IV catheter in place for a prolonged time may increase the risk for clot formation, as can long-term use of peripherally inserted central catheters.

4. Crossing the legs may affect circulation and promote clot formation.

Precaution

A clot can originate in a deep vein in an immobilized patient, especially in the calf or thigh. Avoid massaging patients' legs in a vigorous manner because it can cause blood clots to become dislodged and result in embolization.

PULMONARY HYPERTENSION, SECONDARY

In pulmonary hypertension, the pressure in the pulmonary arteries is higher than normal, but not related to aging or altitude. Primary pulmonary hypertension (with no known etiologic conditions) is rare, but potentially fatal. Many cases of secondary pulmonary hypertension are linked to other conditions or disorders that cause hypoxemia potentially leading to anatomic vascular changes and increased pulmonary resistance in predisposed patients. These include obstructive sleep apnea, obesity, and altered immunologic disorders, as well as chronic pulmonary diseases, such as chronic obstructive pulmonary disease.

Main Symptoms

The presentation of secondary pulmonary hypertension may be obscured by, and similar to, the presentation of the underlying disorders. Potential manifestations include the following symptoms:

- Dyspnea on exertion
- Fatigue and weakness
- Chest pain and signs of hypoxemia, such as altered mental status
- Exertional syncope (fainting)

Many patients may eventually show signs of right-sided heart failure, such as peripheral edema, jugular vein distension (JVD), or ascites.

Selected Nursing Tips

1. Identify patients at high risk for developing pulmonary hypertension; administer appropriate oxygen therapy. Skilled supportive care entails careful observation while carrying out treatment orders to slow the progress of the disease.
2. Monitor the patient's vital signs and ABG analysis for hypoxemia or respiratory acidosis (e.g., hypercapnia); watch for changes in level of consciousness or restlessness and impaired tissue perfusion.
3. Observe the patient's response to oxygen therapy for hypoxemia; report undesirable outcome and adjust the patient care plan accordingly. Correct the underlying causes in collaboration with the healthcare team, such as obstructive sleep apnea.
4. Take measures to maintain optimal fluid status for the patient; check for signs of fluid overload, such as jugular vein distension.
5. Provide patient education regarding prescribed medications and diet. Remind the patient to refrain from overexertion and to obtain adequate rest as needed.

Points to Consider

1. Unlike systemic blood pressure, pulmonary arterial pressure cannot be measured indirectly. Thus, secondary

pulmonary hypertension is not clinically recognizable until the disease progresses to a late stage.

2. Primary pulmonary hypertension is uncommon. For patients with secondary pulmonary hypertension, their prognosis may depend on the severity of the underlying diseases and the alteration of the pulmonary vascular bed.

Precaution

Prevent or treat conditions that can induce hypoxemia, which may initiate the disease process of pulmonary hypertension.

TUBERCULOSIS

Tuberculosis (TB), an infectious disease, is primarily caused by *Mycobacterium tuberculosis*, a bacterium that frequently affects the lungs and is commonly transmitted by the airborne route. This pathogen can be transmitted via sputum or droplets from a patient with active TB as a result of coughing, sneezing, laughing, or talking—that is, the bacteria pass through the respiratory tract of the patient. Transmission may occur after close, frequent, and prolonged contact.

Main Symptoms

Symptoms of TB may be nonspecific, including unexplained weight loss, weakness, night sweats, or low-grade afternoon fever. Hemoptysis (bloody sputum) is largely associated with more advanced TB cases.

Elderly patients may have atypical presentations, such as anorexia, weight loss, or a change in mentality and behavior. Some may have a delayed (or no) reaction to the tuberculin skin test, possibly due to age-related dysfunction of immunologic memory.

Selected Nursing Tips

1. Patients with active TB should be placed in respiratory isolation, staying in a private (possibly negative-pressure) room in which the air is vented to open air outside, as per protocol or requirement.

2. An important nursing role in caring for patients with TB is to educate patients about the medications, including the dosage schedule and side effects. Emphasize the importance of strict adherence to the regimen, preferably watching patients swallow the medications.

3. Ensure adequate nutrition by providing frequent, small, high-carbohydrate and high-protein meals with essential nutrients and vitamins. Supplemental vitamin B_6 is often prescribed if the patient receives isoniazid (INH) to prevent drug-induced neuritis.

4. Stress the importance of getting plenty of fresh air and reporting signs of persistent cough, fever, or hemoptysis, which may indicate recurrence.

5. The proper way to administer an intradermal Mantoux PPD (purified protein derivative) TB test is to hold the syringe with the needle almost parallel to the skin of the person's forearm while inserting the needle. The result is read within 48-72 hours (or as recommended) and recorded as the diameter of the induration (hardened area).

Points to Consider

1. Tuberculosis is often treated with multidrug therapy, such as isoniazid (INH), rifampin (Rifadin), and pyrazinamide (Tebrazid), or a fixed combination of the drugs for many (possibly 6-24) months.

2. A positive Mantoux test may indicate the patient has been exposed to TB or bacilli Calmette–Guérin (BCG) vaccine. In an immunosuppressed patient, however, a negative Mantoux test does not necessarily exclude TB infection, because the patient may not be able to develop an immune response adequate to produce a positive skin test result. The X-ray will show the lesion if it is large enough. A sputum acid-fast bacilli (AFB) smear together with TB cultures can be used to support the diagnosis of tuberculosis. (The lab technique is called "acid-fast bacilli smear" due to the fact that bacilli are not easily stained; once the test is done with a dye, it is

difficult to remove the stain, even with acid alcohol.) *M. tuberculosis* is susceptible to heat and ultraviolet light.

3. Before airborne precautions are discontinued, make sure the required number of consecutive sputum cultures are negative, free of acid-fast bacteria. The patient may still be infected, but the disease is no longer contagious at this point. For TB screening purposes, once an individual has had a positive TB skin test, an X-ray should be used instead of the Mantoux test in later years.

4. Unlike *Staphylococcus aureus*, the TB bacillus is carried in exhaled droplets of patients with an active TB infection, usually not on their personal items. Adhere to respiratory precautions; label all sputum specimens with AFB precautions.

Precautions

1. In addition to being toxic to some organs such as the liver, rifampin may cause reddish-orange discoloration of secretions such as urine, sweat, saliva, or tears, which may stain contact lens. Warn the patient to limit intake of alcohol while on rifampin or INH as instructed by the physician.

2. Long-term isoniazid therapy may cause drug-induced peripheral neuropathy (e.g., a sensation of tingling or numbing), due to vitamin B_6 deficiency. Supplemental pyridoxine (vitamin B_6) is often prescribed to mitigate this effect.

3. Monitor for the signs of adverse effects of antitubercular antibiotics. Streptomycin, an aminoglycoside, may cause nephrotoxicity, ototoxicity, and neurotoxicity, among other side effects. Monitor the patient's serum creatinine and blood urea nitrogen (BUN) level; instruct the patient to report hearing loss and ringing in the ears.

OTHER POINTERS AND CONCERNS

PERTAINING TO ALLERGY

The patient with allergic rhinitis needs to be taught how to use a nasal inhaler to ensure better inhalation. Specifically, the patient should hold one nostril closed while using a nasal inhaler to spray the medication into the other nostril.

Allergic reaction to a contrast medium used for medical tests or procedures may have systemic or local manifestations, including respiratory distress, hypotension, stridor, localized itching, or edema.

Life-threatening anaphylactic reactions and respiratory distress can be caused by latex allergy in susceptible individuals. Before touching patients with hands wearing latex gloves or anything made of latex such as a urinary catheter, make sure the patient is not allergic to latex.

PERTAINING TO BREATHING

Hearing and feeling the air movement from a patient's mouth and nose are more effective ways to determine the patency of an airway than observing the chest rising and falling.

A sitting position, if not contraindicated, may facilitate lung expansion and exhalation in a patient who is experiencing difficulty breathing. This position decreases the abdominal pressure on the diaphragm (the dome-shaped muscle that separates the abdomen from the thoracic cavity).

Upon auscultating rales (crackling) in the base of the lungs, the nurse may ask the patient to take a deep breath or cough. Hypoventilation (reduced rate and depth of breathing) may also be the cause of rales.

Pursed-lip breathing (exhaling through pursed lips for two or three times as long as inhaling) facilitates maximum elimination of CO_2 in patients with COPD. This kind of breathing works by forcing the patient to use the abdominal muscles to keep the air passages open for more complete exhalation.

Cheyne–Stokes respirations are characterized by a period of apnea followed by deep, frequent breathing. These respirations are a serious sign indicating a grave prognosis in adult patients.

Kussmaul's breathing is a deep, rapid, gasping respiration often associated with diabetic ketoacidosis or coma.

PERTAINING TO CARBON MONOXIDE POISONING

Toxicity caused by carbon monoxide can be lethal and requires immediate treatment. Hemoglobin absorbs carbon monoxide much more readily than it absorbs oxygen. In red blood cells, hemoglobin is the iron containing pigment that carries oxygen from the lungs to the tissue cells. When hemoglobin is bound with carbon monoxide, it loses its oxygen-carrying capability. (Pulse oximetry does not provide valid information in patients with carbon monoxide poisoning, because hemoglobin will be saturated with carbon monoxide in this condition.)

Individuals with carbon monoxide poisoning may have altered mental status, as the central nervous system needs a constant and sufficient supply of oxygen to function properly. They may experience headache, weakness, dizziness, and slight confusion. They may also display changes in skin color, ranging from pale and cyanotic to "cherry red."

In addition to carrying out treatment orders, nurses should institute safety precautions to minimize the risks of falls and injuries in patients with carbon monoxide poisoning. Provide fresh air or oxygenation to reverse hypoxia. Loosen constrictive clothing, keep the patient warm, and reduce stimuli to decrease oxygen consumption.

PERTAINING TO (POSTOPERATIVE CARE FOR) NASAL SURGERY

After a patient has undergone nasal surgery, signs of frequent swallowing should prompt the nurse to conduct further examination to rule out the possibility of blood trickling down the throat.

Monitor the patient for signs of ineffective breathing due to possible airway obstruction, resulting from nasal edema or dislodgement of nasal packing. Instruct the patient to avoid activities requiring exertion, such as exercise, vigorous coughing, or straining on defecation, which increase stress on the sutures and the risk of bleeding—the nasal cavity is extremely vascular. The patient may need stool softeners to avoid constipation.

The first step in managing nosebleed (epistaxis) is to have the patient lean forward while sitting to prevent aspiration of blood. Apply pressure by pinching the soft portion of the nose against midline septum to stop bleeding.

After surgery, intermittent cold compresses may be applied to the nose, as appropriate, for its vasoconstriction effect to reduce swelling, bleeding, and pain. Warm, moist compresses may be used later for comfort in the tender area.

PERTAINING TO (SIDE EFFECTS OF) NARCOTICS

One of the many serious side effects of narcotic analgesics (pain pills) is respiratory depression. Assess the patient's level of consciousness as well as the respiration rate as indicated. Patients with a very low respiration rate may need to be roused to enhance their breathing, and to check their oxygen saturation rate and breathing sounds. The practitioner may need to be notified for possible lab or treatment orders.

PERTAINING TO OXYGENATION

Arterial blood gas (ABG) analysis provides measurements of pH and the partial pressures of oxygen and carbon dioxide in arterial blood. These values can be used to assess the blood's acid–base balance and the status of pulmonary gas exchange. ABG analysis is often used to help assess patients' oxygenation as well as help manage their respiratory and metabolic (renal) acid–base balance and their electrolyte status. (The patient's clinical condition has to be taken into consideration concurrently.)

The pH (power of hydrogen) scale is designed to reflect changes in the hydrogen ion (H^+) concentration in a simplified way. (An acid is a substance that releases hydrogen ion when dissolved in solution, while a base accepts it.) When the H^+ concentration increases, the pH value decreases. Comparatively speaking, a blood pH value of 7.2 is more acidic than a pH value of 7.3. The pH of human blood must be maintained within a narrow range, 7.35 to 7.45. When blood pH is below the normal range (pH < 7.35), a problem of acidemia (abnormal acidity of the blood) is present. When blood pH value exceeds 7.45, there is a problem of alkalemia (abnormal alkalinity of the blood).

Partial pressure describes the pressure of a specific gas as part of the total gas mixture. PaO_2 is a measure of the partial pressure exerted by oxygen when dissolved in the arterial blood. $PaCO_2$ is the arterial (partial) pressure of carbon dioxide. CO_2 is produced by cell metabolism when O_2 is consumed for energy; it is excreted by the lungs. (Other acids are excreted in the urine by the kidneys.)

Hypoxemia refers to a state in which the arterial blood oxygen is reduced. Hypoxia refers to a state in which tissues receive an oxygen supply inadequate to maintain normal aerobic metabolism. An increased pulse can indicate the heart's attempt to compensate for such a reduced oxygen supply to the body tissues.

The oxygen saturation level indicates the percentage of hemoglobin saturated with O_2. In most cases, it can be assessed adequately with a pulse oximeter, by applying the probe over a pulsating vascular bed, such as the fingertips or earlobes. A decrease in the oxygen saturation level may be an early indication of respiratory compromise. Unlike ABG analysis, however, pulse oximetry does not provide information on the partial pressure of carbon dioxide.

The lungs are responsible for CO_2 removal, with the effectiveness of this process being determined by alveolar ventilation. Increased $PaCO_2$ (hypercapnia) and respiratory acidosis usually result from ineffective breathing (hypoventilation). The initial assessment findings in such a case may include a compensatory increase in the rate and depth of respiration, as well as altered mental status.

Hyperventilation due to anxiety (or resulting from the body's compensatory mechanism when the sympathetic nervous system is activated) may cause excessive loss of CO_2, leading to respiratory alkalosis. This condition manifests with symptoms such as tingling around the mouth and dizziness. Having the patient breathe into a paper bag to rebreathe the expired carbon dioxide may offset respiratory alkalosis to some degree.

Remind the patient who is receiving oxygen to be aware of the risks of fire associated with oxygen use: Oxygen supports the combustion process. If the patient is receiving low-dose oxygen and an item nearby catches on fire, first make sure the patient is not in immediate danger, and then turn off the oxygen.

PERTAINING TO SUCTIONING

Suctioning removes oxygen as well as secretions, and it may also cause trauma to the mucosa. Suctioning should be performed on an as-needed basis. It is important not to apply suction while a catheter is being inserted. Intermittent suction should be applied only when a catheter is being withdrawn in a swirling motion.

Properly hyperoxygenate the patient before and after a suctioning procedure, as the depletion of oxygen from the suction may trigger dysrhythmias. Stop suctioning and re-oxygenate the patient as indicated.

After suctioning, auscultate the patient's breath sounds to evaluate the effectiveness of the efforts to clear the airway.

An unconscious patient is unable to maintain a clear airway independently. In caring for a comatose patient, suction as indicated to promote airway clearance.

CHAPTER 4

Neurologic Issues

The neurosensory system is the body's communication network, which transmits impulses between different parts of the body. The neurons—the basic nerve cells—are the structural and functional units of the nervous system. To understand complex neurologic disease processes, it is beneficial to review some facts and terms related to the neurosensory system first.

The nervous system consists of two subsystems:

- The central nervous system (CNS)
- The peripheral nervous system (PNS)

The CNS includes the brain and spinal cord. The brain contains three major components:

- The cerebrum, which consists of two cerebral hemispheres. The left hemisphere is responsible for language control, and the right hemisphere has greater control over nonverbal perceptual functions.
- The cerebellum, which is involved in controlling and coordinating skeletal muscle movements (in concert with other brain structures).
- The brain stem, which is composed of the midbrain, pons, and medulla oblongata.

The cerebrum controls voluntary movements and conscious thought, including the limbic system, which is associated with emotion. The cerebral hemispheres are divided into the frontal, parietal, temporal, and occipital lobes:

- The frontal lobe controls cognition and voluntary movement. Broca's area in the frontal lobe is responsible for expressive speech.
- The temporal lobe is concerned with receptive speech as well as bodily, visual, and auditory input.
- The parietal lobe integrates spatial information.
- The occipital lobe is associated with vision, processing sight stimuli.

The cerebellum functions to maintain trunk stability and coordinate voluntary movement. The brain stem, which connects to the spinal cord, consists of the midbrain, pons, and medulla oblongata. These vital centers are associated with management of respiration, vasomotor, and heart function.

The PNS consists of 12 pairs of cranial nerves; 31 pairs of spinal nerves, which contain both sensory and motor fibers; and portions of the autonomic nervous system. The 12 pairs of cranial nerves are numbered according to the order in which they emerge from the brain:

Cranial Nerve Number	Cranial Nerve Name	Selected Functions
I	Olfactory	Sense of smell
II	Optic	Visual perception
III	Oculomotor	Eye movement muscles, pupil changes, lens accommodation
IV	Trochlea	Eyeball movement
V	Trigeminal	Facial motor and sensory innervation
VI	Abducens	Lateral eye movement
VII	Facial	Facial muscle movement and expression, salivation

Cranial Nerve Number	Cranial Nerve Name	Selected Functions
VIII	Vestibulocochlear	Sense of hearing and equilibrium
IX	Glossopharyngeal	Gag reflex, swallowing, salivation, sense of taste
X	Vagus	Regulate heart rate and respiration, visceral sensations; parasympathetic innervation of thoracic and abdominal organs
XI	Accessory	Movement of head, neck, and shoulder
XII	Hypoglossal	Tongue movement for speech and swallowing

The spinal nerves are named by their location. There are 8 cervical spinal nerves, 12 thoracic spinal nerves, 5 lumbar spinal nerves, 5 sacral spinal nerves, and 1 coccygeal spinal nerve, corresponding to the spinal vertebrae.

The autonomic nervous system (ANS) regulates the involuntary functions of cardiac and smooth muscle as well as the glands. It consists of two divisions—sympathetic and parasympathetic—which counterbalance each other to maintain homeostasis (equilibrium).

The sympathetic division reacts to stress by releasing neurotransmitters or hormones. For example, norepinephrine is a neurotransmitter that acts on adrenergic receptors to produce the body's physiological "fight or flight" responses. A sympathetic response usually results in an increase in blood pressure (BP), pulse, systemic circulation, and mental alertness, and, simultaneously, a decrease in secretions, digestion, and urine output.

Comparison of Effects	Sympathetic Nervous System	Parasympathetic Nervous System
Heart beat rate and strength	↑	↓
Pupils	Dilation	Constriction
Sweat	↑	
Saliva secretion	↓	↑
Urinary sphincter	Contraction	Relaxation
Hairs	Contraction with goose pimples	
Adrenal medulla secretion	↑ Epinephrine	
Pancreatic secretion of insulin	↓	↑
Peristalsis	↓	↑
Liver (glycogenolysis)	↑ increased glucose level	
Blood vessels (α receptors)	Constriction	
Blood vessels (β receptors)	Dilation	

The parasympathetic division primarily dominates in non-stressful situations. Its main neurotransmitter acetylcholine (ACh) acts on cholinergic receptors to induce its effects, including conserving energy, decreasing heart rate, and increasing peristalsis and glandular/gastrointestinal secretions. ACh is rapidly degraded by the enzyme acetylcholinesterase.

There are two types of basic neural cells:

- Neurons
- Neuroglia or glial cells

The neurons are responsible for impulse initiation and conduction. Each neuron has three parts: a cell body, an axon, and one or more dendrites. Many axons are covered with a myelin sheath, an insulating white lipid substance. Destruction of the myelin sheath is often the cause of neurologic problems or diseases, such as in multiple sclerosis. The glial cells nourish and support the neurons.

DISORDERS AND CONDITIONS

ALZHEIMER'S DISEASE

Alzheimer's disease (AD) is a common form of dementia related to the degenerative structural changes of the brain; it brings progressive, irreversible loss of intellectual functions. AD may be caused by a complex combination of factors that contribute to the progression of the disease, including aging, deficiencies of neurotransmitters such as acetylcholine, head trauma, environmental factors, and genetic or nongenetic inducers.

Main Symptoms

- Loss of recent memories, which interferes with the patient's daily routines
- Subtle personality changes due to ongoing loss of neurons
- Speech disturbances
- Cognitive impairment and inability to perform purposeful acts, recognize familiar persons and objects, or communicate via writing

Symptoms are usually first noticed by family members. As the disease advances, patients tend to completely lose the ability to govern their own affairs and to perform self-care routines. Some tend to wander away from home or get lost and become combative.

Selected Nursing Tips

1. It is important to arrange for the patient to have a safe living environment with close supervision.
2. Measures should be taken to prevent complications, including injuries, malnutrition, dehydration, and infection.

Encourage the patient to engage in proper exercise to maintain mobility.

3. Nurses should show empathy and support for the caregivers as well as the patient. Build an effective communication system to facilitate family adjustment to the patient's increasing need for care.

Points to Consider

1. Some medications—such as donepezil (Aricept), a cholinesterase inhibitor that increases cholinergic effects—may slow cognitive decline in some patients with AD. Be sure not to change their dosage without the physician's direction. Overdose may cause cholinergic crisis, evidenced by symptoms such as increased salivation, respiratory depression, and hypotension. Avoid stopping cholinesterase inhibitors suddenly, as abrupt discontinuation can trigger behavior problems.

2. Memantine (Namenda) is used to reduce the actions of chemicals contributing to the symptoms of Alzheimer's disease. Among its many possible side effects, it may cause dizziness and headache, affecting performance that requires alertness. Ensure the patient's safety and adequate fluid intake.

3. Antihistamines and tricyclic antidepressants such as amitriptyline (Elavil) should be avoided because of their significant anticholinergic effects.

4. Aging is a risk factor for AD, but dementia is not part of normal aging. The clinical diagnosis of AD is made mainly by exclusion, although decreased neurotransmitter levels and physiological changes in the brain can be found in some tests. Definitive diagnosis is often confirmed by examination of the brain at autopsy. Treatment research is ongoing and new diagnostic technologies are under development.

Precaution

Patients with AD may wander and get lost. They may also exhibit sundowning behavior, in which they become more confused during the evening. Risk of injury is the greatest concern with such patients. Patients with AD should wear an ID bracelet to facilitate their return home in case they wander away.

AMYOTROPHIC LATERAL SCLEROSIS (LOU GEHRIG'S DISEASE)

In amyotrophic lateral sclerosis (ALS), also known as Lou Gehrig's disease, patients have defective motor neurons, which are replaced with fibrous tissues. The result is impaired impulse conduction caused by hardening of the anterior and lateral columns of the spinal cord—hence the term "lateral sclerosis." The term "amyotrophic" refers to the muscular atrophy and wasting away associated with this disease. ALS typically causes progressive muscle degeneration, but usually does not affect the muscles that control the rectum and bladder. The exact cause of ALS has not yet been identified.

Main Symptoms

- Progressive muscular weakness and ataxia (incoordination)
- Increasing difficulty in walking, speaking, swallowing, or breathing, leading to total debilitation (resulting from disuse syndrome)
- Almost no cognitive changes in most patients

Selected Nursing Tips

1. Nursing care should promote independence to the greatest extent possible. Institute measures to reduce the risk of aspiration, falls, and other injuries. Assist with passive range-of-motion exercises and with obtaining supporting devices, such as a walker or wheelchair.

2. Reduce the risk of aspiration; keep oxygen and suction equipment readily available for emergencies.
3. Nursing interventions may include referring the patient and the family to support groups, and helping the patient have an advance directive in place as the disease progresses.

Point to Consider

Be aware of new medications, such as riluzole (Rilutek), which is being studied for its effects on slowing the deterioration of the motor neurons in ALS.

Precaution

Potential respiratory problems are the most serious concern in patients with ALS. The nurse should first administer oxygen when dyspnea (difficulty in breathing) is noted.

BELL'S PALSY

Bell's palsy often results from unilateral inflammation of the seventh cranial (facial) nerve, causing one-sided facial-muscle weakness or paralysis and distorted facial appearance. Most patients have a complete recovery and rarely experience recurrence. The exact cause of Bell's palsy is unknown.

Main Symptoms

- Initially, pain behind the ear or numbness or stiffness on the affected side
- Facial expression distortion and unilateral facial weakness
- Inability to smell, frown, close the eye, or show teeth on the affected side
- Possible mouth drooping, drooling, and difficulty chewing

Selected Nursing Tips

1. Reassure the patient that Bell's palsy is not the same as a stroke and that most patients will achieve recovery without residual effects.

2. Advise patients to prevent eye dryness or injury by using artificial tears, closing the paralyzed eyelid manually, or wearing eye patches or glasses if prescribed.
3. Implement supportive measures as instructed by the healthcare provider; measures may include using lukewarm moist cloths, gentle upward facial massage, or facial exercises appropriately to stimulate the return of functions and prevent muscle atrophy. Advise patients to avoid exposure to cold or drafts.

Points to Consider

1. The diagnosis of Bell's palsy is made primarily by exclusion.
2. Viral infection, such as herpes simplex, may be implicated in this condition's etiology. If corticosteroids are used, they must be gradually tapered off.

Precautions

1. Measures must be taken to prevent eye (cornea) injuries.
2. Have the patient sit up to eat as a means to prevent aspiration related to difficulty swallowing on the affected side.

BRAIN TUMORS

Primary brain tumors arise from tissues and structures within the brain. Secondary brain tumors are more common, resulting from metastasis of tumors located elsewhere in the body.

Main Symptoms

Presenting symptoms depend on the location and growth rate of the tumor. Clinical findings may include the following symptoms:

- Progressive cognitive dysfunction, involving memory problems or personality changes
- Persistent headache
- New onset of seizures
- Other signs of increased intracranial pressure (ICP), such as nausea, projectile vomiting, and abnormal respiration rate and depth

A nonmalignant tumor grows slowly, often involving no cerebral edema. It may produce no symptoms until it becomes quite large.

Selected Nursing Tips

1. Minimize environmental stimuli. Implement seizure precautions and management plans to prevent injury.
2. Use a calm and reassuring approach; establish a well-structured routine. Provide redirection if the patient is confused.
3. Performing a comprehensive assessment to be used as baseline data is important.
4. Postoperatively, prevention of increased ICP—a potential complication of craniotomy—is essential. Position the patient's head properly and raise the head of bed as per protocol to aid in breathing and decreasing cerebral edema. If fluids are restricted, monitor for signs of dehydration.
5. Closely watch for changes in neurologic status. Avoid Valsalva maneuver if possible, such as straining to have bowel movements, which can increase ICP.

Points to Consider

1. Promptly report sudden unilateral pupil dilation with loss of reaction to light, which may suggest serious complications.
2. Monitor the patient's intake and output to detect postoperative complications involving the pituitary gland, such as diabetes insipidus (DI) or syndrome of inappropriate antidiuretic hormone (SIADH).
3. The Glasgow Coma Scale is used to assess a patient's reaction to stimuli. Eye-opening, verbal responses, and motor responses are solicited from the patient to determine his or her level of consciousness. It is especially useful for monitoring the patient's changes in mental status during an acute phase. However, it cannot replace an in-depth neurologic assessment.

Precautions

1. Abnormal respiration rate and depth may suggest increased ICP, which should be addressed.
2. Clear, colorless drainage from the eyes, ears, or nose may be leakage of cerebrospinal fluid (CSF); this finding should be reported and leaking CSF ruled out.

CEREBRAL ANEURYSM

Cerebral aneurysm refers to a dilation of cerebral arterial walls resulting from a weakened area in the cerebral artery. The exact cause of aneurysms is not clear. Possible contributing factors may include degenerative changes due to aging; atherosclerosis, which may result from deposits of cholesterol, lipids, and calcium in the arterial walls; and other conditions, including hypertensive vascular disease, head injury, congenital defects, or degenerative changes due to advancing age. Rupture of a cerebral aneurysm is often the cause of hemorrhagic stroke.

Main Symptoms

An aneurysm may remain asymptomatic until it is about to rupture. The rupture is often abrupt and without warning, with the patient possibly experiencing the following symptoms:

- Severe headache and blurred vision if conscious
- Change in level of consciousness and restlessness due to increased intracranial pressure, resulting from the additional blood in the cranium
- Nuchal rigidity, nausea, vomiting, and back and leg pain
- Seizure and coma

Selected Nursing Tips

1. Maintain a patent airway. If appropriate, slightly elevating the head of the bed or proper positioning may facilitate pulmonary drainage and prevent airway obstruction.
2. Monitor IV infusions to avoid fluid overload and prevent increased ICP.

3. Any stimuli—such as nicotine, television, or reading—that can increase blood pressure or ICP should be avoided to prevent recurrent bleeding. Lighting should be dimmed and the environment kept quiet.

4. Advise the patient to avoid exertion (e.g., pushing, lifting, and even blowing the nose or coughing) and limit daily activities to a minimum.

5. Monitor arterial blood gas (ABG) levels and vital signs. Avoid taking a rectal temperature, as vagus nerve stimulation may cause cardiac dysrhythmia.

6. Provide patients with a high-bulk diet and stool softeners as ordered to prevent constipation or straining, which may increase the patient's risk for rebleeding (especially if analgesic codeine is prescribed). Rectal fecal impaction checks should be avoided in such patients, as vagus nerve stimulation may potentially cause cardiac dysrhythmia or arrest.

Point to Consider

Life-threatening events that may be associated with cerebral aneurysm include increased ICP, rebleeding, vasospasm, and hemorrhagic stroke, all of which may lead to altered brain function.

Precaution

After the initial bleeding episode, the patient is at risk for rebleeding; a ruptured intracranial aneurysm may result in hemorrhagic stroke, bleeding into the brain tissue.

CEREBRAL PALSY

Cerebral palsy (CP) comprises a group of nonprogressive neuromuscular disabilities. The term "palsy" denotes that some degree of paralysis is present. CP may result from defects or trauma possibly sustained near the time of birth. Probable causes include anoxia (lack of oxygen), hemorrhage, and other damages to the central nervous system.

Main Symptoms

- Spastic muscle movement, muscle weakness, and tendency toward contractures
- Involuntary movement and speech difficulty
- Incoordination, tremor, and ataxia (defective muscle coordination)

Patients often fail to achieve developmental milestones and have other problems, such as hyperactivity or short attention span.

Selected Nursing Tips

1. Collaborate with other healthcare staff to promote patients' self-care abilities to achieve the maximum independence (or near-normal life skills) within their physical limitations.
2. Ensure the provision of adequate nutrition, and institute safety precautions to reduce the risk for complications and injuries.
3. Render all care in an unhurried way. Provide support and guidance for families of chronically handicapped patients.
4. Advocate good prenatal care to avoid premature birth and prevent cerebral palsy.

Points to Consider

1. Causes of most cerebral palsy cases are unknown, but prematurity or perinatal trauma may play a role in its development. The disease is not contagious; no cure is yet available.
2. Muscle deterioration may occur due to a lack of use (disuse atrophy). Starting physical therapy early, soon after the diagnosis is made, may promote muscle strength.

Precaution

Measures should be taken to avoid contractures with muscles fixed in a rigid position.

CONCUSSION

Concussion, or mild traumatic brain injury, involves a temporary interruption of brain function, after a person sustains a head injury without confirmed structural damage. It may or may not cause a brief loss of consciousness.

Cerebral contusions and lacerations are more serious injuries, involving bruising and tearing of the brain tissues, respectively. Loss of consciousness is often present with these injuries, frequently associated with stupor or confusion.

Secondary injury may evolve over time after the initial (primary) injury, possibly resulting from insufficient supply of nutrients and oxygen to the brain cells.

Main Symptoms

Symptoms of concussion vary depending on the severity of the impact, but may include the following:

- Amnesia (a loss of memory) for what occurs surrounding the traumatic events
- Headache, irritability, and lethargy
- Dizziness
- Visual defects, such as diplopia or blurred vision
- Nausea and vomiting

Neurologic deficits may appear later. Although concussion usually resolves over time, some patients with prior concussions or head injuries may develop a progressive neurologic problem.

Selected Nursing Tips

1. Treat all patients with head injury as if a cervical spinal injury is present. Proper head and neck immobilization is indicated unless confirmed otherwise. Immobilize, assess, and stabilize the patient per protocol.
2. For a patient with suspected cervical spinal injury, follow the emergency care guidelines and maintain a patent

airway. Hyperextension of the neck, as created by the usual head tilt/chin lift maneuver, may worsen a cervical spinal injury.

3. Monitor the patient with head injury for signs of increased ICP resulting from possible bleeding or edema; the initial sign may be an altered level of consciousness (LOC), including being slightly drowsy with slurred speech. Closely monitor the patient for signs of respiratory compromise and intervene as indicated.

4. The family should be instructed to monitor the patient closely and wake up a sleeping patient at intervals. Signs of confusion, problems with speech or arousal, vomiting, severe headache, and one-sided weakness should be promptly reported to the practitioner.

5. When unconscious patients regain consciousness, the nurse should reorient them to time, person, and place.

Points to Consider

1. Severe head injury involving the posterior pituitary gland may cause temporary antidiuretic hormone (ADH) deficiency, leading to diabetes insipidus or other problems. When the patient has a urine output much larger than fluid intake, the signs of colorless urine and low urine specific gravity may raise suspicion of the onset of DI.

2. A patient with head or neck injury may have damage to the spinal cord, potentially with subsequent neurologic symptoms.

Precaution

Soon after sustaining a mild concussion, the patient should not be given strong narcotics. Sedative or analgesic (pain-relieving) effects may alter the level of consciousness and mask the severity of the injuries.

ENCEPHALITIS: ARBOVIRAL

Encephalitis is characterized by an acute inflammation and swelling of the brain tissue. This condition can be attributed to various etiologies, such as infection with herpes simplex virus, fungi, and other pathogens. Arthropod-borne encephalitis is often caused by viruses, mostly transmitted via mosquito or tick bites.

Main Symptoms

Most types of viral encephalitis have similar symptoms:

- Sudden onset of fever
- Headache, confusion, and drowsiness
- Nausea or vomiting because of increased intracranial pressure
- Stiff neck due to meningeal irritation
- Seizures and coma

Many cases of West Nile encephalitis involve mild flu-like symptoms. Some cases, however, may lead to serious neurologic disorders, such as meningitis.

Selected Nursing Tips

1. Frequently assess the patient's neurologic function, especially during the acute phase of the disease. Take precautions against potential falls or seizures to prevent injuries.
2. Patients on bed rest should be encouraged to turn or change positions often and to increase fluid intake, as appropriate, to prevent complications induced by immobility, such as altered elimination or deep vein thrombosis. Fluid overload, which may increase the risk for cerebral edema, should be avoided.
3. Monitor for signs of neurologic deficits and dehydration secondary to nausea, vomiting, or fever. Intervene immediately if the patient becomes lethargic or hard to rouse.
4. Supportive care and assistance should be rendered as needed.

Points to Consider

1. Nursing management of encephalitis, including West Nile virus infection, is generally supportive to alleviate symptoms.

2. Advanced age is a risk factor for encephalitis. Take steps to prevent insect-borne infection, including installing screen windows and removing standing water (where mosquitoes might hatch).

3. Some antiviral agents, such as acyclovir (Zovirax), may be effective against herpes encephalitis if used early in the course of the disease.

4. Providing a calendar or a clock in the room may help orient a confused patient.

Precaution

The patient's respiratory and circulatory status are of primary concern. Monitor for signs of changes of vision, behavior, or sleep patterns. Initially, intensive care may be necessitated.

GUILLAIN–BARRÉ SYNDROME

Guillain–Barré syndrome (GBS) is a potentially fatal form of polyneuritis although most patients can anticipate spontaneous and complete recovery, albeit over months or years. This disease may be an immunologic response, resulting in segmental nerve demyelination (loss of the fat-like insulating substance around the nerve axons), and subsequently leading to impaired peripheral neurotransmission and rapid muscle weakening or paralysis.

Main Symptoms

Manifestations of GBS may vary, depending on the severity and the nerve affected. The ascending type of GBS often starts from the distal (farthest) lower extremities, with muscle weakness then progressing upward. Symptoms may include the following:

- Paresthesia (numbness and tingling)
- Reduced muscle tone and reflexes
- Pain or muscular ache

Nerve demyelination may potentially cause serious consequences, including inability to swallow or clear secretions and cardiovascular instability.

Muscle atrophy is not usually present when the diagnosis is made (due to GBS's rapid onset) and cognitive function is commonly not affected.

Selected Nursing Tips

1. The patient's increased hoarseness should be reported due to the likelihood of airway and respiratory compromise.
2. Monitor the patient closely for changes in vital signs, lab results, and heart rhythm. Be vigilant for signs of respiratory failure resulting from paralysis affecting the diaphragm.
3. If patients experience muscle aches or cramps, analgesics (to alleviate discomfort) may be needed before range-of-motion exercises or repositioning.
4. Liquids may need to be thickened before serving, because patients with dysphagia are more likely to aspirate thin fluids.
5. Provide meticulous care to prevent complications, including infection, cornea irritation and drying, and problems secondary to altered elimination or immobility.

Point to Consider

Guillain–Barré syndrome often occurs following an episode of respiratory or gastrointestinal viral infection, or other precipitators; it is characterized by muscle weakness that progresses rapidly. Therapy (e.g., IV immune globulin or plasmapheresis) may be used in some cases to directly influence or alter the peripheral-nerve myelin antibody level.

Precautions

1. Guillain–Barré syndrome is a medical emergency; keep emergency equipment, such as an intubation kit, readily available. Respiratory support and ventilator assistance may be necessary in some cases. In addition, continuous

electrocardiographic (ECG) monitoring may to be needed to reduce the risk of complications caused by patients being immobilized or on a ventilator, especially when patients are receiving therapies to decrease circulating antibody levels, such as plasmapheresis.

2. Aspiration precautions should be initiated, due to the potential loss of patients' gag reflex and possible drooling.

HEADACHE

Headache is a common physical discomfort and complaint; it is a symptom of an underlying disorder or condition. It may be attributed to a multitude of factors arising from both intracranial or extracranial sources, ranging from the stress response, environmental stimuli, head or neck trauma, muscle tension, vasodilation, and hypoxia to organic diseases or a combination of these factors.

Headache can be classified into many types and subtypes based on various factors and characteristics. It can also be described as primary with no identifiable cause or secondary to other conditions. Some patients can experience headaches of different types simultaneously.

Main Symptoms

Migraine headache is one of the more serious forms of headache, and may occur with or without aura. The manifestations of migraine with aura can proceed through different phases with different presentations. During an acute attack, the headache may be severe and incapacitating, with patients experiencing unilateral throbbing pain, irritability, sensory dysfunction, or sweating accompanied with nausea and vomiting or photophobia of varying duration.

Tension-type headache may be intermittent, described as a feeling of pressure with photophobia or phonophobia (fear of sound or noise).

Cluster headaches, lasting different lengths of time, may be excruciatingly painful. They may occur repetitively (or even in succession), with periods of remission lasting for months or years.

Some headaches may be associated with inflammation, such as cranial arteritis, and possibly visual disturbances. Symptoms may vary widely because of the different etiologies and underlying conditions.

Selected Nursing Tips

1. Help the patient identify the causes or triggers of his or her headaches, and implement strategies for preventing the recurrence of headache.
2. Obtain a thorough medical history. Provide medication information and individual education based on the characteristics and type of headache to reduce anxiety and stress; suggest beneficial lifestyle or habit modifications.
3. Evaluate the responses and effectiveness of ongoing treatment regimens through close monitoring; encourage avoidance of known triggers, including certain medications. Migraines may be precipitated by certain foods containing nitrates, those containing monosodium glutamate (MSG), and aged cheeses, among others, in susceptible individuals.
4. Nonpharmaceutical management should be employed when possible, but pain-relieving medications should not be withheld or delayed.

Points to Consider

1. Observance of a consistent and regular schedule for daily activities, including relaxation, exercise, meals, and sleep, may be helpful in preventing recurrent episodes of headache.
2. Stress reduction should be recommended and implemented where stress is unavoidable.
3. Sumatriptan (Imitrex), an antimigraine medication, may be prescribed for treatment of acute migraine headache or cluster headache. This agent relieves headache by causing

cranial blood vessels to constrict. Note the maximum daily dosage, dose interval, and contraindications for sumatriptan, including ischemic heart disease and renal impairment. Follow instructions regarding drug interactions, dosing, and administration to prevent severe adverse effects, including tremor, agitation, reduced respiration, and seizures. Tablets should be taken whole (with a full glass of water) and should not be crushed or split.

Precaution

Persistent headache may require medical evaluation to rule out organic diseases, such as brain tumor, stroke, hypertension, and meningitis, even though most headache is not caused by a serious disorder.

HUNTINGTON'S DISEASE/CHOREA

Huntington's disease (HD), a hereditary neurologic disease, is associated with an excess of dopamine, possibly resulting from a deficiency of some neurotransmitters, such as acetylcholine. It causes symptoms opposite to those of parkinsonism, including abnormal and excessive involuntary facial, limb, or body movements (chorea) and cognitive deterioration. As with Parkinson's disease, the pathologic process for HD involves the basal ganglia and the extrapyramidal motor system.

Main Symptoms

- Chorea with abnormal and excessive involuntary facial, limb, or body movements
- Depression, delusion, and restlessness
- Impaired speech, chewing, and swallowing abilities

Huntington's disease is progressively debilitating. Patients eventually lose the physical and mental capability to walk and take care of themselves, though they often retain their muscle strength.

Selected Nursing Tips

1. Provide patients with a safe living environment that is as comfortable as possible, and focus nursing care on patients' needs given their impaired capabilities.
2. Assess and minimize patients' risks of malnutrition, choking and aspiration, injuries, and infection.
3. A nursing care plan may encompass enlisting interdisciplinary efforts, addressing strategies to manage symptoms, such as depression or dementia, chorea, swallowing difficulties, ambulation limitations, and bowel/bladder incontinence. It may also include making appropriate referrals to community organizations where psychosocial support is available.

Point to Consider

Patients and families may benefit from regular nursing palliative and protective care, although there is no effective treatment to halt the relentless progression of the disease process.

Precaution

Clinical manifestations may not be evident until the patient reaches reproductive age; carriers can be identified through genetic tests. Refer affected families to genetic counseling, because this disease is hereditarily transmitted.

INTRACRANIAL PRESSURE, INCREASED

Increased intracranial pressure (ICP) is a major nursing concern while caring for patients with neurologic disorders. Many disorders can cause ICP to rise, leading to compression and ischemia when the compensatory mechanism ultimately fails. The increased ICP may result from an increase in any of the brain's three essential volume components: brain tissue, blood, and cerebrospinal fluid.

A variety of factors normally influence ICP, including changes in abdominal or thoracic pressure (posture, coughing, straining), temperature, and blood gases. Balanced volume is usually maintained by the body's autoregulation processes and compensatory mechanisms, such as dilation or constriction of the blood vessels and changes in the CSF volume in the brain. The brain's capacity to adjust is limited, however. When the brain fails to adapt to the changes, decompensation (ischemia and infarction) occurs.

Main Symptoms

- Altered mental status, the earliest symptom of increased ICP—initially a subtle change in the level of consciousness, such as a decrease in the level of attention or a change in orientation
- Unexpected or projectile vomiting, possibly related to cranial pressure change
- Vision change
- Headache
- Symptoms of cerebral ischemia, including blurred vision or syncope (fainting), resulting from inadequate cerebral perfusion

The neurons of the cerebral cortex need a constant supply of oxygen and glucose for cerebral functions, and are highly sensitive to decreased cerebral blood flow (CBF).

The characteristic signs of decompensation (ischemia or infarction) associated with increased ICP are known as Cushing's triad. This trio of symptoms is considered a grave sign:

- Increased systolic blood pressure and pulse pressure (the difference between the systolic and diastolic readings)
- Bradycardia (decreased heart rate) with a bounding pulse
- Bradypnea (decreased respiration rate)

Selected Nursing Tips

1. Initial nursing interventions to reduce ICP may include positioning the patient properly and keeping neutral functional alignment to facilitate venous drainage from the

head and lower ICP. Avoid extreme hip flexion to prevent an increase in intra-abdominal pressure. Neurologic checks are implemented per protocol.

2. Irritating stimuli should be minimized and the environment kept calm and quiet. Suctioning, coughing, sneezing, straining, and Valsalva maneuvers should be discouraged or prevented, if feasible. Keep suctioning to a minimum per protocol in duration (after administering oxygen properly).

3. Space nursing care activities to minimize transient increases in ICP. Prevent fever to reduce the risk of cerebral edema; address concerns to prevent infections and complications.

4. Take measures to prevent constipation. Monitor the patient who is on fluid restriction for signs of dehydration, such as poor skin turgor, dry mucous membranes, and decreased urine output and blood pressure.

5. If the patient has been prescribed mannitol (Osmitrol), an osmotic diuretic, monitor for signs of dizziness or fluid and electrolyte imbalances. If a steroid drug is prescribed to treat cerebral edema or inflammation, monitor the patient for signs of infection or gastrointestinal (GI) bleeding and other steroid-related side effects. Make sure the steroid medication is not discontinued abruptly, as adrenal crisis can occur. Note that steroids can also mask the symptoms of infection.

Points to Consider

1. Cerebral edema is often a contributing factor for increased ICP.

2. If there are no other causative conditions, a sluggish pupil reaction to lights and unequal, dilated, or fixed pupils may also be signs of increased ICP, suggestive of decompensation.

Precaution

Observe patients who have sustained head trauma for signs of increased ICP. Administering sedatives or pain medication before the diagnosis is made can obscure symptoms of increased ICP.

MENINGITIS

Meningitis refers to an inflammation of the lining (meningeal tissues) surrounding the brain and spinal cord; it often represents a complication of another infection or condition. The causative agents can be bacteria, viruses, and other organisms or substances. Bacterial meningitis is a medical emergency, and early treatment is key to successful patient outcomes.

Main Symptoms

Common clinical findings in bacterial meningitis include the following signs and symptoms:

- Fever, chill, and malaise
- Nausea, vomiting, and severe headache
- Stiff neck (nuchal rigidity) with positive Kernig's and Brudzinski's signs
- Signs of increased ICP
- Possible purplish discoloration (petechiae) on the face or extremities
- Seizures

The clinical presentation of viral meningitis is similar to that of bacterial meningitis, but the symptoms are often less severe.

Selected Nursing Tips

1. Assess the patient's level of consciousness first and often. Watch for signs of deterioration and increased ICP, such as visual disturbance with cranial nerve involvement.
2. Administering ordered drugs—such as ceftriaxone (Rocephin), vancomycin (Vancocin), cefuroxime (Ceftin), and others (according to etiology, severity, and sensitivity)— is critical in combating and managing bacterial meningitis.

Check the IV site frequently to prevent complications such as infiltration and phlebitis; monitor for signs of the side effects of the medication.

3. Measures must be taken to reduce fever, including using Tylenol and Motrin alternatively if so prescribed. Fever can increase cerebral edema and the risk of seizures.
4. Maintain adequate hydration, but avoid fluid overload due to the danger of cerebral edema.
5. Efforts should be made to minimize environmental stimuli; place the patient on seizure precautions.
6. To relieve the discomfort of photophobia, keep the room dark or offer the patient a cool cloth to be placed over the eyes if desired.
7. Droplet precautions should be instituted, including wearing isolation masks and gloves while in close contact with the patient.

Points to Consider

1. The incidence rate of meningococcal meningitis is higher in people with respiratory or ear infections, who are debilitated, or who are living in a crowded environment.
2. Early detection and treatment are essential. Vaccination may offer some protection against this infectious disease.
3. Tobacco use is one of the risk factors for developing and spreading meningitis, because it increases respiratory secretions and droplets.

Precautions

1. Before the patient is discharged, a hearing test may be necessary, due to possible damage to the nerve responsible for hearing.
2. The mortality rate is especially high in patients with untreated bacterial meningitis. Symptoms of septicemia may include high fever, purpuric lesions, shock, and manifestations of disseminated intravascular coagulation (DIC).

MULTIPLE SCLEROSIS

Multiple sclerosis (MS), a progressive degenerative disorder, commonly affects the myelin sheaths in the brain and spinal cord. In MS, myelin may be replaced by scar tissue, forming sclerotic plaques in multiple areas of the central nervous system. As a result, nerve impulse conduction is impaired. Patients sometimes experience repetitive exacerbations and spontaneous remissions, as the myelin can regenerate itself.

Main Symptoms

During MS exacerbations, nerve impulse conduction and muscle innervation are inadequate. Manifestations vary in their severity and duration, and depend on the nerves affected. Patients may develop signs of sensory or motor impairment and emotional problems:

- Sensory abnormalities (e.g., sensation of numbness or tingling, pins and needles, or other paresthesia or neuropathic pain)
- Visual abnormalities (e.g., patchy blindness, blurred vision, or double vision)
- Hearing impairment (e.g., tinnitus—subjective ringing in the ears)
- Muscular dysfunction (e.g., weakness, spasticity, balance problem, or paralysis)
- Bowel or bladder problems if the associated nerves are affected
- Emotional instability with generally intact cognition

These problems may not be present during remission, when the myelin has regenerated.

Selected Nursing Tips

1. Direct nursing care toward maintaining the patient's self-care ability and usual function for as long as possible.

2. Advise the patient to plan daily activities to avoid stress, fatigue, or heat, which may exacerbate MS symptoms. Moderate exercise is often therapeutic; discourage patients from participating in strenuous exercise that raises body temperature.

3. Advise patients to test the temperature of bath water and avoid direct contact with hot appliances; patients with MS frequently experience sensory loss, which can increase their risk for burn/thermal injury.

4. Provide adequate hydration to reduce the risk of urinary tract infection (UTI) secondary to a neurogenic bladder/ urinary retention and to aid in bowel elimination.

5. If the patient's condition permits, high fiber and fluid intake will help establish a bowel program.

6. Remind patients to routinely inspect their skin for injuries or pressure points; patients' motor-sensory loss poses a threat that skin injuries and pressure sores will go unnoticed.

Points to Consider

1. The exact cause of MS is a subject of ongoing research; its course is unpredictable and highly individualized.

2. The cause of death is often related to infective complications.

Precaution

Institute preventive measures, as patients may be at risk for complications, some resulting from altered sensory and motor functions (e.g., aspiration due to dysphagia and falls due to ataxia and others, such as infections, due to medications and lowered immunity).

MYASTHENIA GRAVIS

In myasthenia gravis ("grave muscle weakness"), transmission of nerve impulses to the voluntary muscles is impaired. This condition may possibly result from an autoimmune response, in which antibodies attack a portion of the acetylcholine receptor sites, leading to fewer receptors available for muscle stimulation. Fluctuating muscle weakness is a characteristic feature of myasthenia gravis.

Main Symptoms

Initial manifestations include the following signs and symptoms:

- Eye muscle weakness with ptosis (drooping of eyelid) and diplopia (double vision)
- Fluctuating weakness involving other muscles, including those of the neck or extremities

Symptoms may be exacerbated by stress, overexertion, or exposure to excessive heat, and relieved by rest.

Myasthenic crisis, an exacerbation and a life-threatening complication of the disease, is often precipitated by medication changes, infection, or other conditions. It is characterized by severe muscle weakness involving the muscles used for chewing or breathing with symptoms such as the following:

- Dysarthria (defective speech)
- Dysphagia (difficulty swallowing)
- Severe respiratory distress

In cholinergic crisis (caused by overmedication with cholinesterase inhibitors), patients may also have respiratory distress, severe muscle weakness, and dizziness.

Selected Nursing Tips

1. Nurses should emphasize the importance of taking medication on time to reduce the risk of drug-related crises. Teach patients about the potential adverse effects of missing doses or overdoses of medication.
2. Advise patients to take their medication before meals to improve muscle strength for proper chewing.

3. Instruct patients to pace their daily activities to prevent fatigue.
4. Educate patients to avoid stress or exertion, including exposure to excessive heat or crowds, which may exacerbate their symptoms.

Points to Consider

1. Anticholinesterase/cholinergic drugs, such as neostigmine (Prostigmin) and pyridostigmine (Mistinon), inhibit destruction of acetylcholine and facilitate transmission of nerve impulses, which promote normal muscle function in patients with myasthenia gravis. As the disease progresses, these drugs may become less effective, requiring medication adjustment.
2. The Tensilon test may be used in diagnosing myasthenia gravis or differentiating between myasthenic and cholinergic crisis. A dose of an anticholinesterase/cholinergic drug such as edrophonium (Tensilon) may produce improvement in a patient with myasthenia gravis or who is in myasthenic crisis, but leads to worsening signs in a patient in cholinergic crisis. Respiratory support and an antidote such as atropine should be available during the test, as cardiorespiratory depression can occur.

	Myasthenic Crisis	**Cholinergic Crisis**
Causes	Exacerbation or following a precipitating event	Possibly overdose of cholinergic drugs
Test results using a dose of a short-acting anticholinesterase, such as edrophonium (Tensilon)	Muscle strength improves	Muscle weakness worsens

Precautions

1. Patients in myasthenic crisis usually require constant monitoring and need vigorous respiratory support in the hospital setting.
2. Tensilon is not used to treat myasthenia gravis because of the short-acting nature of this medication.

PARKINSON'S DISEASE

Primary Parkinson's disease (PD), a progressive neurologic movement disorder, is associated with decreased levels of dopamine due to degeneration of neurons in the substantia nigra of the brain. Consequently, there is an imbalance between two neurotransmitters: dopamine and acetylcholine. Dopamine is essential in maintaining normal functions of the extrapyramidal motor system, including movement and posture control.

Main Symptoms

- Tremor at rest—possibly the first sign before rigidity becomes obvious
- Rigidity with increased muscle tone
- Bradykinesia (extremely slow movement) or difficulty initiating movement
- Mask-like face and drooling
- Stooped posture, with head and trunk bent forward and legs flexed
- Shuffling gait

Selected Nursing Tips

1. Teach patients that medication should be taken at the scheduled time, so that the effectiveness of drug therapy can be evaluated accurately. Improvement of muscle rigidity is a desired effect of the drug therapy.
2. Encourage patients to exercise in the morning when rested, or after taking medication, which helps patients have a better range of motion.

3. Patients may find it difficult to initiate movement or get up from a seated position. Recommend that they choose higher, firmer chairs and an elevated toilet seat, or rock back and forth to assist themselves in standing up.

4. Offer frequent, small, and soft meals to minimize fatigue and prevent aspiration. Provide a balanced diet to overcome problems related to nutrition and elimination.

5. Provide clothing with Velcro fasteners and the like, so as to promote self-care and functional abilities to the greatest extent possible.

6. Praise patients for their perseverance in performing daily living activities.

Points to Consider

1. Secondary PD, which includes extrapyramidal syndrome (EPS), can result from different causes, including chemical poisoning and medications, such as the antipsychotic medication chlorpromazine (Thorazine) or the antiemetic metoclopramide (Reglan). Prolonged use of such medications may induce tardive dyskinesia (involuntary movements of face, trunk, and arms).

2. Carbidopa/levodopa (Sinemet), a dopamine precursor, increases the concentration of dopamine in the brain. Carbidopa makes more levodopa available to be transported into the brain. Taking the medication with food can minimize its potential to cause GI upset. Warn the patient that the medication may cause harmless darkening of urine or sweat, and that its effect may be delayed from weeks or even several months after initiation of the therapy.

3. When patients are prescribed some antiparkinson agents, such as ropinirole (Requip) or pramipexole (Mirapex), warn patients against postural hypotension; patients should get up from a lying or sitting position slowly. Hallucinations may also occur, especially in elderly patients.

Precautions

1. Patients' unsteady gait poses a risk for falls. Maintaining a safe environment is an important aspect of care.
2. Parkinsonian crisis may be associated with sudden withdrawal of medication or emotional trauma.

RABIES

Rabies (hydrophobia), an acute viral infection, is primarily transmitted via the saliva from the bite of a rabid (often unprovoked) animal, or from bats without a direct bite. The virus can also be spread by casual contact with scratches, secretions, or airborne droplets from infected mammals. The salivary glands and pharyngeal muscle are often affected, resulting in abnormal salivation and laryngeal spasm at the sight or sound of water.

Main Symptoms

After a period of incubation, the patient typically experiences tingling, numbness, itching, or pain at the bite site, in addition to flu-like symptoms. Neurologic symptoms may include agitation, hypersalivation with characteristic frothing of the mouth, and hydrophobia (abnormal fear of water). Other serious symptoms, such as nuchal rigidity, apnea, and coma, may lead to respiratory and cardiovascular collapse.

Selected Nursing Tips

1. Vigorously wash the bite with soap and water for at least 10 minutes to cleanse the wound.
2. Seek medical treatment as soon as possible.
3. Treat the wound or bite, and administer medication or vaccine (post-exposure prophylaxis) as ordered.

Point to Consider

Encephalitic rabies is often fatal; its incidence is greatly reduced in areas where vaccination is implemented.

Precautions

1. Rabies can be carried in any warm-blooded mammals, including bats, skunks, foxes, and raccoons. Prevent rabies by vaccinating pets and avoiding wild animals.
2. Unless proven otherwise, suspect rabies in the victim of an unprovoked animal bite; presumption of exposure is important because rabies is often lethal.

SEIZURES/EPILEPSY

In seizure, a sudden abnormal electrical discharge of neurons in the brain interferes with normal function, including motor, sensory, autonomic, or psychological activities. Epilepsy refers to recurrent seizures that are often due to an underlying disorder. Various terms are used to describe seizures having different characteristics. There is a seizure threshold for everyone in general population.

Main Symptoms

In a tonic–clonic seizure, the patient may lose consciousness or fall; this event is followed by a tonic phase (stiffening of the body) and then a clonic phase (jerking of the extremities). An absence (petit mal) seizure may present as a vacant stare for a few seconds, often without being noticed. In complex partial seizures, repetitive purposeless activities may be present, including facial grimacing, patting, and lip-smacking.

Selected Nursing Tips

1. In most cases, seizures last a few seconds to a few minutes, and they are usually self-limiting. If a seizure lasts longer than a few minutes, or if continuous seizures occur in rapid succession, emergency medical care should be sought; there is often a protocol for such cases, or an individual doctor's order may be in place. The consequences of seizures can be serious because of patients' brief loss of consciousness during these episodes.

2. The duration of a seizure should to be accurately timed from its start to its end and well documented.

3. The nursing priority during and after a seizure is to keep patients safe, protecting them from injury. Nothing should be placed in the patient's mouth during a seizure.

4. Seizure assessment should include documenting the duration and characteristics of seizure activities, and the patient's condition before, during, and after seizures.

5. Take measures to prevent complications, including aspiration, injury, and hypoxia. After a seizure, the patient is at risk for aspiration due to possible drooling; a side-lying position may facilitate drainage of oral secretions. Have suction equipment in place in case it is needed.

6. When assessing vital signs in patients with seizure disorder, avoid taking their temperature orally. Other precautions should be taken as indicated on a case-by-case basis.

Points to Consider

1. Some patients may have an aura before losing consciousness. An aura refers to a warning sign or symptom experienced by the patient before a seizure, such as a certain smell, vision, or sensation.

2. After a seizure episode, the patient may experience post-ictal drowsiness or somnolence (trance or sleepiness); take necessary precautions to ensure the patient's safety.

3. The side effects of phenytoin (Dilantin), a commonly prescribed anticonvulsant, may include overgrowth of gums, drowsiness, and toxicity, among others. Good oral hygiene may prevent gingivitis.

4. Other medications often prescribed to control seizure activities include valproic acid (Depakote), topiramate (Topamax), lamotrigine (Lamictal), levetiracetam (Keppra), and carbamazepine (Tegretol). To maintain their therapeutic effects, serum drug levels are monitored at regular intervals as required. Watch for their side effects;

implement seizure precautions, including providing a safe, quiet environment for patients.

Precautions

1. Prolonged seizure is a medical emergency. Abrupt discontinuation of anticonvulsants may precipitate a life-threatening episode of persistent seizure.
2. Seizure medication should be administered exactly as prescribed on a regular basis so as to maintain drug levels within safe and therapeutic ranges.

SPINAL CORD INJURY

The spinal cord serves primarily as the pathway for the transmission of sensory impulses to the brain and motor impulses from the brain. It also mediates defecation and urination reflexes as well as stretch reflexes.

Spinal cord injuries (SCI) are major health problems. They may result from various causes, including motor vehicle accidents, falls, and other traumas or injuries. Areas of flexibility such as the neck and lower back are more vulnerable to such injuries.

Main Symptoms

The presentations of SCI may depend on the impact of external force and the severity or location/level of the injury. The patient may or may not have acute pain in the back or neck. A cervical injury is more likely to cause tetraplegia (quadriplegia—paralysis of all four extremities), whereas injuries at the thoracic or lumbar level may result in paraplegia (paralysis of the lower body and of both legs).

Selected Nursing Tips

1. Suspect spinal cord injury in patients who have suffered direct trauma and who complain of pain in the head, neck, or back, unless SCI has been ruled out. Follow the emergency management protocol. Properly handling such injuries

and avoiding disturbing the patient's body alignment are of paramount importance, as any twisting movement can irreversibly exacerbate spinal cord damage.

2. Initiate early treatment to minimize secondary injuries resulting from ischemia, hypoxia, edema, and bleeding that stem from the initial trauma; such care is essential to prevent further damage.

3. Monitor patients for signs of neurologic changes, such as altered skin sensation or muscle strength. These changes may be caused by pressure on the spinal cord due to edema or shifting bone fragments.

4. After acute spinal injury, some patients may experience the neurologic syndrome known as "spinal shock"—that is, loss of reflexes/sensations and motor control below the injury level. This complication should be reversed as quickly as possible to prevent permanent paralysis.

5. Autonomic dysreflexia (hyper-reflexia) is a life-threatening condition, which often occurs in patients with high-level SCI after the resolution of spinal shock (with the return of reflexes); it can be the sympathetic nerves' over-response to noxious stimuli. Acute symptoms typically include the following:
   - Extremely high blood pressure
   - Intense headache
   - Bradycardia (slow heart rate)
   - Flushed face and diaphoresis (often of the forehead)

   To rule out autonomic dysreflexia, it is important to take the blood pressure and pulse of a patient with high-level SCI who is complaining of headache. The causative stimulus below the injury level should be identified and removed. Sitting the patient up (to possibly lower the blood pressure), assisting the patient in emptying the bladder or eliminating a fecal impaction, removing support hose or skin irritation/pressure, and managing blood pressure may be indicated. The practitioner should be contacted if the patient's symptoms are not relieved with such interventions. To prevent the recurrence of autonomic dysreflexia (even years after the initial injury), institute measures to establish regular elimination routines and avoid pressure on the lower extremities.

6. Patients with spinal cord injury should be told to avoid caffeine, which can contribute to bladder spasm, resulting in reflex incontinence. Maintaining skin integrity is also a nursing priority.

Points to Consider

1. The spinal cord injury cannot be accurately evaluated until the spinal shock resolves.
2. The sensation of spasticity felt by a patient with spinal shock may indicate the return of reflexes, signaling possible recovery.
3. A support system is especially important to patients with spinal cord injuries. Patients afflicted with paralysis will need the support of the family; significant others should be involved in education related to the discharge instructions.

Precaution

Trauma patients who report back pain are better moved by trained personnel to prevent additional spinal cord damage.

STROKE, ISCHEMIC

Stroke, or cerebrovascular accident (CVA), is also known as "brain attack," signifying the urgency of this problem. In ischemic stroke, patients experience a sudden onset of neurologic deficits, resulting from inadequate blood supply to an area of the brain. This condition requires immediate medical interventions to prevent the loss of functional neurons and brain cells. Stroke may be described with different terms according to its etiology, characteristics, or other criteria. Although there are some similarities between "ischemic" stroke and "hemorrhagic" stroke, the medical or nursing management approaches to these conditions differ in certain aspects.

Temporary neurologic deficits resulting from a brief period of insufficient blood flow and oxygen in the brain are known as transient ischemic attacks (TIAs). TIAs rarely cause permanent neurologic deficits. When the blood flow returns to normal, the TIA-related symptoms may disappear. They can, however, signal an increased risk for CVA in some patients.

Main Symptoms

In ischemic stroke, patients experience dysfunction of voluntary motor control on one side of the body; such hemiplegia may reflect upper motor neuron damage on the other side of the brain, because many motor and sensory nerves cross from one side of the body to the other. The sudden-onset symptoms, which vary with the severity of the stroke, include the following:

- Numbness and weakness of the face, arm, or leg, particularly on one side of the body
- Loss of vision, confusion, slurred speech, and difficulty understanding words
- Loss of coordination
- Severe headache and change in mental status or cognitive function
- Seizure or coma

Other neurologic deficits associated with stroke may include the following conditions:

- Alexia: inability to read
- Agraphia: inability to write
- Aphasia: inability to speak
- Dysphagia: difficulty swallowing
- Dysphasia: difficulty understanding speech or communicating verbally

Selected Nursing Tips

1. Being familiar with the warning signs of a stroke can make a big difference in the likelihood of saving the patient's

brain tissue or even his or her life. Activate the emergency system immediately at any sign of a stroke such as slurred speech, confusion, and one-sided weakness or sensory change. The American Stroke Association suggests that the mnemonic FAST may serve as a reminder of the stroke symptoms and the fast response required: **f**acial drooping, one **a**rm drifting downward, **s**peech changed or slurred, "**t**ime is essential." A fast response may minimize the stroke damage or potentially reverse a dire disease process.

2. Initially maintaining the patient on NPO (nothing by mouth) status is usually necessary until the stroke has stabilized. Ensure that suction equipment is available at all times, in case the patient loses the gag reflex and his or her level of consciousness decreases.

3. Provide ongoing care and education. Assess the neurologic deficits according to the nursing recommendations and take measures to prevent complications. When a patient has one-sided muscle flaccidity, a sling or splint may be used as ordered to support the affected limb and prevent deformity.

4. In a patient with residual dysphagia after a stroke, liquids should be thickened to prevent aspiration. Patients should not be fed when their gag reflex is absent.

5. The following signs of aspiration should be reported:
    - Coughing or choking while eating
    - Difficulty breathing
    - Low O_2 saturation (arterial hemoglobin oxygen-saturation level obtained using a noninvasive pulse oximeter)
    - Elevated temperature

6. Blood pressure should not be obtained from the side of the patient that is paralyzed.

7. When providing oral care to patients who have suffered a stroke, position the patient on his or her side to minimize the risk of aspiration.

8. Place the patient's personal-care items on the over-bed table on the patient's intact side and approach the patient

from this visual field. The patient with hemianopsia (loss of half of the visual field) should be reminded to turn his or her head to scan the entire environment, including the missing vision field.

9. Before discharge, patients should be assessed for the risk of recurrent CVA and encouraged to take measures to lower these odds, including following the medication regimen, monitoring and controlling blood pressure, and making necessary lifestyle changes.

10. Counsel patients on ways to maintain skin integrity, including inspecting the skin carefully daily or shifting weight at regular intervals.

Points to Consider

1. When assessing a patient with thrombotic or embolic stroke (not hemorrhagic stroke) for possible administration of tissue plasminogen activator (t-PA), the nurse should first try to determine the time of onset of the current stroke, so as to weigh the potential benefits of thrombolytic therapy against the bleeding risks. Patients receiving t-PA during the window established by the drug's manufacturer or evidence-based guidelines after the onset of a stroke may have a better outcome. Other contraindications for t-PA therapy should also be ruled out, including head injury.

2. It is crucial to control the patient's blood pressure after providing treatment for ischemic stroke because cerebral hemorrhage is the major side effect of thrombolytic therapy.

3. Stroke prevention is the best approach; advocate a healthy diet, an appropriate level of daily exercise, maintenance of normal weight, and maintenance of normal blood pressure (or normal blood sugar level in patients with diabetes). Smoking and heavy drinking increase the risk of stroke.

Precaution

It is important to treat and manage atrial fibrillation and hypertension, as they increase the risk of stroke. Atrial fibrillation may predispose patients to clot formation, leading to embolization and stroke. Uncontrolled high blood pressure is a risk factor for hemorrhagic stroke.

TRIGEMINAL NEURALGIA

Trigeminal neuralgia (formerly known as tic douloureux) results from a disorder of the trigeminal cranial nerve (cranial nerve V). It is characterized by recurrent excruciating unilateral facial pain or twitching, and periodic remissions.

Main Symptoms

The typical feature of this disorder is a repetitive, unilateral "shock-like" pain in the lips, gums, cheek, or side of the nose. Patients may exhibit grimacing, twitching, blinking, or tearing during a brief acute attack—hence the term "tic."

Many factors may cause minimal stimulation affecting the nerve in the trigger zones, precipitating acute pain. Potential triggers include the following events:

- A draft of air
- Washing the face
- Light touch or yawning
- Brushing the teeth or shaving
- Ingesting cold or hot food

Selected Nursing Tips

1. Help the patient identify precipitating factors and minimize triggering stimuli.
2. Advise the patient to chew soft food on the unaffected side, and to avoid temperature extremes, either on the face or in food.
3. Monitor the patient for signs of anxiety and depression; employ proper interventions and make appropriate referrals.

Points to Consider

1. Trigeminal neuralgia is relatively benign but may be traumatic for patients.
2. If the patient is receiving carbamazepine (Tegretol), ask the patient to immediately report fever, sore throat, and easy bruising. These symptoms may be early clinical evidence of toxicity, requiring reevaluation of the medication regimen.

Precaution

Institute measures to prevent depression, dehydration, and malnutrition, because patients may avoid socializing and neglect hygiene or nutrition as a result of this disorder.

CHAPTER 5

Sensory Issues

The eyeball has three major layers. The external layer consists of the sclera and cornea. The sclera is also known as "the white of the eye." The cornea is the transparent, avascular, most anterior portion of the eyeball; it is the main refracting surface, which bends the light rays that enter the eye and helps focus them on the retina. To keep it healthy, the cornea obtains oxygen from the air dissolved in the tears.

The middle, vascular layer of the eye is the uvea, which consists of the iris, ciliary body, and choroid. The iris is the colored part of the eye. Its small round center is the pupil, through which light enters the eye. The pupil constricts when it is used for near vision or when bright light enters the eye; it dilates for far vision or in a dim environment. Behind the pupil and iris is the biconvex, transparent lens; it can change its shape to better focus light rays on the retina. (This kind of "accommodation" is controlled by the ciliary body.)

The third inner layer of the eye is the retina, which lines the inside of the eyeball, and extends and forms the optic nerve. The retina converts an image perceived by the eye into a form that the brain can process as vision. The macula, an area of the retina, receives light from the center of the visual field and provides the greatest visual acuity.

The aqueous humor is produced by the ciliary body. This watery fluid, which provides nutrients and oxygen to this area, is constantly formed and drained to maintain a relatively constant intraocular pressure (IOP). Increased IOP often results from inadequate drainage or absorption of the aqueous humor, potentially causing ischemia of the neurons of the eye and damage to the optic nerve.

The conjunctiva is a transparent mucous membrane that lines the inner surface of the eyelids and also covers the sclera. Thus, it forms a "pocket" under each eyelid.

DISORDERS AND CONDITIONS OF THE EYE

CATARACTS

An opacity or cloudiness of the lens of the eye is referred to as a cataract. Cataracts are one of the common causes of vision loss. The development of cataracts is mostly age related, with this condition being more prevalent in older adults.

Cataracts usually develop bilaterally at varied rates. The exception is traumatic or congenital cataracts, which may remain unilateral or stationary.

Main Symptoms

- Painless, progressively decreased or blurred vision
- Sensitivity to glare in bright lights, which worsens at night when pupils dilate
- In severe cases, the black pupil becoming milky white

Selected Nursing Tips

1. Suggest palliative measures, including using visual aids or driving only in daytime, until surgery is indicated to correct functional visual impairment.
2. After a cataract is surgically removed, some patients may be prescribed an eye shield to be worn at night for protection, along with certain activity restrictions, such as avoiding bending or stooping, which may increase IOP.

Point to Consider

Cataracts can also arise secondary to exposure to chemicals, ultraviolet (UV) light, or radiation. In addition, they may stem from other conditions or trauma to the eyes. Certain drugs, including corticosteroids (even long-term topical use), are associated with the development of cataracts.

Precautions

1. After surgery, patients should avoid coughing or straining, if possible. Take measures to prevent constipation in these individuals.
2. One of the potential complications of cataract surgery is retinal detachment; advise them to immediately report symptoms such as seeing new floaters and flashes of light, which may potentially signal the development of retinal detachment.

CONJUNCTIVITIS

The conjunctiva is a transparent mucous membrane that covers the inner surface of the eyelids and extends over the sclera (the "white" of the eye). In conjunctivitis, commonly described as "pink eye," there is an infection or inflammation of the conjunctiva. Conjunctivitis can be caused by bacteria, viruses, allergy, or other irritants.

Main Symptoms

Patients with bacterial conjunctivitis may experience purulent drainage, redness (due to subconjunctival blood vessel congestion), irritation, or tearing of their eyes.

Patients with viral conjunctivitis may report tearing, foreign body sensation, or redness. Viral conjunctivitis is usually self-limiting, and antiviral eye-drops are largely ineffective in treating this condition.

Selected Nursing Tips

1. Advise the patient to avoid or remove the source of eye irritation or infection, and emphasize the importance of hand washing after touching the eyes and nasal secretions.
2. Avoid contaminating the tip of the bottle when instilling antibiotic eye-drops. Use individual towels or disposable tissues to contain the condition.
3. Remind people working near chemical irritants to wear safety glasses as a precaution.

Points to Consider

1. Conjunctivitis is highly contagious. Sharing the patient's personal items, such as towels or reading glasses, should be avoided.
2. Chronic conjunctivitis may be caused by degenerative changes to the eyelids.

Precaution

Thorough handwashing is essential before and after having contact with a patient with conjunctivitis, so as to prevent the spread of any infectious agents.

GLAUCOMA

Glaucoma is characterized by a slow loss of retinal neurons, often related to increased intraocular pressure resulting from an imbalance in the formation and absorption/drainage of the aqueous humor (fluid) in the structures of the eyes. Some patients with glaucoma may have normal IOP. Glaucoma is largely a disease of aging, but often has a strong genetic component.

If untreated, glaucoma may cause optic nerve damage, leading to peripheral vision loss or blindness. The decreased blood supply to the neurons of the eyes can also contribute to optic nerve deterioration.

In open-angle glaucoma, which accounts for the majority of the cases, the patient has neuronal degeneration, but open drainage angles. In closed-angle glaucoma, the elevated eye pressure commonly results from a defect (impaired aqueous outflow) in the drainage mechanism. An acute closure event in these patients is an ophthalmic emergency, and often has a rapid onset. It may also be triggered by situations in which the pupil stays in a partially dilated state long enough to cause an acute rise in IOP, resulting from factors including drug-induced mydriasis (abnormal pupil dilation from topical eye preparations or systemic drugs), emotional upset, or darkness.

Secondary glaucoma may result from the conditions that block the drainage channel in some way, including trauma or an inflammatory process.

Main Symptoms

There are no early symptoms of open-angle glaucoma. When the patient begins to notice peripheral vision loss, the disease is already at an advanced stage. (The intraocular pressure tends to be above the normal range or high for the individual.) Initially, this type of glaucoma affects peripheral vision, leading to painless, progressive narrowing of the visual field.

During an angle-closure event, the patient may report colored haloes around lights, blurred or foggy vision, or occasionally severe eye pain.

Selected Nursing Tips

1. Teach the patient to report eye pain and have regular eye-pressure checks. Seriously increased intraocular pressure is an ophthalmic emergency, which should be treated as soon as possible to prevent nerve damage.
2. Instill the prescribed eye-drops, such as latanoprost (Xalatan) or bimatoprost (Lumigan), exactly as prescribed. If a patient has more than one kind of eye-drops, allow some time (at least 10–15 minutes) between the administrations of different medications

to prevent one drug from being diluted by another. To prevent the drug from being systemically absorbed, slightly apply pressure over the corner of the eye near the nose (medial canthus) immediately after the eye-drops administration.

3. The desired effect of therapy for glaucoma is to control intraocular pressure, often by facilitating the clearing or draining of fluid from the eyes.

4. Advocate glaucoma screening for early detection and encourage prevention for people over 35 years of age or who have a family history of glaucoma.

Points to Consider

1. With early detection and appropriate treatment, including long-term medication therapy to maintain IOP within normal limits, blindness from glaucoma is largely preventable.

2. Patients with angle-closure glaucoma should be advised to avoid darkness, emotional stress, use of anticholinergic medications, and other factors that cause the pupils to dilate and IOP to increase.

Precaution

If IOP is not properly controlled, blindness may result from optic nerve damage related to high IOP compressing the nerve.

MACULAR DEGENERATION

Degeneration of the macula (an area of the retina) is often associated with aging and can result in irreversible central vision loss. The dry, or atrophic, form is characterized by a slow and progressive painless vision loss. The wet, or exudative, form is often more severe, with a rapid onset of acute visual impairment. Contributing factors may include genetic predisposition, long-term exposure to UV light, cigarette smoking, and other eye conditions. Nutrition may play a role in slowing the progression of this condition.

Main Symptoms

Patients may have distorted vision or blind spots in central visual field. Initially, straight lines become wavy or bent, possibly in one eye. Over time, progressive central vision decline may result in functional blindness.

Selected Nursing Tips

1. Advise patients to use optical visual aids, such as magnifying glasses or large-print reading material. Better lighting may help patients with macular degeneration to cope with their gradual vision loss.
2. Educate patients to have routine eye exams, and to monitor and report vision changes. The ophthalmologist may recommend using Amsler grids (or other tests) to detect sudden onset of distortion of vision.
3. Refer patients to low-vision service counseling to help them adjust to the inevitable lifestyle changes.

Points to Consider

1. Patients with age-related macular degeneration may experience serious vision loss, but do not always progress to total blindness.
2. Some nutrients or vitamins, such as beta-carotene and certain vitamins, have been studied for their possible effect in lowering the risk of developing this condition. Consultation with a healthcare provider is recommended.

Precaution

Ensure environmental safety through means such as open walkways or other forms of assistance.

RETINAL DETACHMENT

Retinal detachment (RD) refers to the separation of the retina—the sensory portion of the eye, which is the innermost layer of the eye and extends to form the optic nerve—from the underlying epithelium, which causes fluid to collect between the two layers. The detached area may rapidly expand, unless contact between the two layers is reestablished promptly. The neurons of the retina may die because of a lack of blood supply, resulting in permanent vision loss.

Risk factors for retinal detachment include the following conditions:

- Older age
- Severe myopia (nearsightedness)
- Eye injury
- Diabetic retinopathy
- Family history, often associated with myopia

Main Symptoms

Retinal detachment is painless. Some patients may experience the following symptoms:

- Seeing floaters, dark spots, or bright flashing lights in the visual field
- Feeling the sensation of having a shadow, ring, or curtain in the vision

Selected Nursing Tips

1. Arrange for the patient to be seen by an ophthalmologist right away.
2. Preoperatively, instruct patients to refrain from strenuous activities and head movements that increase the risk of further detachment. Presurgery teaching should also include possible postoperative positions and prevention of complications.
3. Postoperatively, the patient may be required to assume a position that brings the retina in contact with the underlying layer to reestablish the blood supply to the retina—for instance, sleep on the abdomen—for a period of time as instructed by the surgeon.

Point to Consider

If not treated in time, the retinal tear, although often localized, can extend to involve the entire retina.

Precaution

Any patient with suspected retinal detachment should be seen by an ophthalmologist without delay.

ANATOMIC POINTERS: EARS

The ear is a sensory organ that has two primary functions: hearing and balance (equilibrium). The main structures of the ear include the external ear, the middle ear, and the inner ear.

The external ear consists mainly of the auricle (pinna) and external auditory canal. The auricle collects sound waves and sends the vibrations into the external auditory canal. The tympanic membrane (eardrum) separates the external ear and the middle ear. The function of the external and middle portions of the ear is to conduct and amplify sound waves received from the environment. Air conduction refers to sound conducted over the air-filled external and middle ear by vibration of the tympanic membrane and auditory ossicles. Hearing problems associated with these two areas may result in conductive hearing loss, affecting the patient's perception of or sensitivity to sounds.

The auditory (or eustachian) tube connects the middle ear with the nasopharynx; the mucous membrane lining the middle ear extends from the nasal pharynx via the auditory tube. The inner ear is partially responsible for hearing and balance, which rely on very complex mechanisms.

DISORDERS AND CONDITIONS OF THE EAR

HEARING LOSS

Hearing impairment is a prevalent form of disability, which can directly affect individuals' quality of life. Conductive hearing loss commonly results from impaired transmission of sounds through the air in conditions such as external ear disorders (e.g., impacted cerumen) and middle ear disease (e.g., otitis media).

Sensorineural hearing loss often results from impaired function of the inner ear or the acoustic nerve (the eighth cranial nerve). Causative factors may include aging, ototoxicity, Ménière's disease, or other serious systemic diseases, such as bacterial meningitis. In this condition, the ability to hear high-pitched sounds or to understand speech may be affected. Exposure to intense loud sounds or prolonged environment noise can cause sensorineural hearing loss. Such hearing loss is common and becomes permanent after the initial repair or restoration period is complete, owing to possible structural damage to hair cells in the organ of Corti, a structure of the cochlea in the inner ear that turns mechanical energy into neural activity and differentiates sounds into various frequencies.

Hearing loss resulting from impairment within the central auditory system (the pathway from the inner ear to the brain) may cause individuals to have difficulty in understanding the meaning of words that are heard.

Functional hearing loss may be psychogenic and nonorganic without detectable structural changes. It is also possible for people to have mixed types of hearing loss.

Main Symptoms

Early signs of hearing loss may include the following:

- Tinnitus
- Preference for higher sound volume and cupping the hand around the ear
- Speech that is uncharacteristically loud (in some types of hearing loss) or soft (often in conductive hearing loss because patients hear their own voice)
- Personality change, such as being uninterested and inattentive in group activities

Often, the person with hearing impairment is not sufficiently aware of the gradually developing hearing problem and may not seek hearing assistance.

Selected Nursing Tips

1. Many people refuse to wear hearing aids for various reasons, including self-consciousness. Take patients' attitude and behavior into consideration when counseling individuals with hearing impairment to ensure a more effective conversation or better persuasion.
2. Educate patients about avoiding loud noises to prevent noise-induced hearing impairment and acoustic trauma. Warn about the danger of using foreign objects, such as cotton swabs, to clean the ear canal to prevent impacted cerumen from damaging the eardrum.
3. Advocate wearing protective ear devices, such as foam ear inserts or earphones, in a dangerously noisy environment as a preventive measure.
4. Be aware of and watch for the side effects of ototoxic medications.
5. Employ strategies to enhance communication with hearing-impaired individuals, such as talking into a less affected ear and using helpful gestures or visual aids; identify patient-specific methods to ensure more effective communication.
6. When conversing with an elderly individual with hearing difficulty, speak distinctly in a relatively low tone.

Points to Consider

1. Recommend audiometric hearing screening and medical assistance to at-risk individuals, including older patients. For patients with sensorineural hearing loss, hearing aids may be ineffective in correcting their deficits.
2. Many occupational or recreational pursuits may increase the risk for hearing impairment, such as carpentry or loud music.

3. A quiet environment is in general more conducive to rest and peace of mind, especially to patients who are acutely ill; keep the noise level to a minimum for patients at rest. Loud, persistent noise may cause increased adrenalin secretion, leading to increased blood pressure.

Precaution

Some medications, such as aminoglycosides and aspirin, are ototoxic, especially when ineffective renal excretion causes patients to have increased serum drug levels. Furosemide (Lasix) is a diuretic that may potentially cause ototoxicity (e.g., tinnitus, vertigo, or deafness), particularly in patients with renal disease; make sure not to administer it at a rate exceeding the specified limit.

MÉNIÈRE'S DISEASE

Ménière's disease (endolymphatic hydrops) manifests with symptoms caused by an inner ear disorder possibly associated with an abnormal accumulation of inner ear fluid (endolymph), which distorts the system. The exact cause of this disorder remains unknown. Although not life-threatening in nature, the sudden episodic vertigo can be disabling, causing falls or injury.

Main Symptoms

Patients may experience recurrent attacks of vertigo with an incapacitating rotational sensation, dizziness with tinnitus (a subjective ear ringing) or a roaring sound, and painless fluctuating hearing loss. The onset of vertigo is often sudden, causing immobility or loss of balance, accompanied by symptoms such as nausea, vomiting, nystagmus (rapid involuntary eye movements), or headache.

Selected Nursing Tips

1. Patients should be advised to get up slowly to maintain their balance, avoid sudden position changes, and turn the entire body to turn the head so as to prevent vertigo.

2. Help patients minimize environmental stimuli, stress, and fall-related risks.

3. Reassure patients that Ménière's disease is not life threatening when safety measures are in place.

Points to Consider

1. If an antihistamine drug, such as meclizine (Antivert) or hydroxyzine (Atarax), is prescribed for vertigo, warn the patient of its potential side effects, including drowsiness and dry mouth.

2. The exact cause of Ménière's disease remains unknown, but it often occurs secondary to infection, fluid imbalances, or major stressors. Smoking and excessive intake of caffeine-containing fluids and salty foods should be avoided.

Precaution

Patient safety is a priority; keep the bed in a low position and provide a safe living environment.

OTITIS MEDIA (MIDDLE EAR INFECTION)

Otitis media (OM) refers to an infection of the middle ear, often secondary to an upper respiratory infection or other inflammatory process (possibly related to obstruction or dysfunction of the eustachian tube). When treated early, acute OM usually has a good prognosis. Prolonged fluid accumulation in the middle ear cavity may result in chronic otitis media and serious complications, potentially including conductive hearing loss.

Main Symptoms

The manifestations of OM vary with the severity of the condition, but may include the following signs and symptoms:

- Pain unrelated to the movement of the external ear
- Fever or flu-like symptoms, such as sneezing or coughing
- Headache (more likely in an acute case) and dizziness
- Vomiting

- Purulent discharge from the ear when the eardrum spontaneously ruptures in severe cases
- Diminished hearing

Selected Nursing Tips

1. Instruct the patient to complete the full course of the prescribed antibiotic therapy to reduce the risk of developing drug resistance.
2. Suggest appropriate intermittent use of warm compresses to alleviate pain. Warmth may dilate the blood vessels in the ear, and promote the reabsorption of fluid.
3. Stress the importance of not getting fluid in the ears.
4. Otitis media often results from an upper respiratory infection or occlusion of the auditory tube; prevent chronic ear infection by promptly treating a respiratory infection or acute OM.

Point to Consider

Given that the mucous lining of the middle ear is anatomically connected to the pharynx via the auditory (eustachian) tube, infectious organisms can enter the middle ear from the nose and throat, and migrate internally. Infants and young children are more susceptible to OM, because the eustachian tube is shorter and straighter in children than in adults.

Precautions

1. Patients with OM should be advised to temporarily avoid airplane trips or diving due to the rapid pressure changes associated with those activities.
2. Patient teaching should include reporting an abrupt relief of pain or pressure, which may indicate perforation of the tympanic membrane; this membrane protects the middle ear from the external environment. Repeated eardrum perforations with extensive scarring can cause hearing loss.

CHAPTER 6

Endocrine Issues

The endocrine system plays a vital role in integrating body functions and maintaining the body's internal homeostasis (dynamic equilibrium) in concert with other systems.

The endocrine glands release hormones (chemical substances) directly into the blood. These hormones bind to their specific cellular receptors in a kind of "lock-and-key" mechanism to influence the target tissue. Secretions are interrelated and interdependent. The overproduction or underproduction of certain hormones will eventually have a serious impact on health, affecting homeostasis.

Major endocrine glands that secrete hormones are the pituitary, thyroid, parathyroid glands, adrenal glands, the pancreas, and the reproductive glands. The hypothalamus primarily controls the secretions of pituitary hormones. The pituitary gland is frequently referred to as the master gland because it secretes some hormones, such as thyroid-stimulating hormone (TSH) and adrenocorticotropic hormone (ACTH), which influence the hormone-secreting actions of the other endocrine glands. Nervous system activity associated with pain, emotions, and stress can also influence the secretion of some hormones. In addition, some other body organs, such as the kidneys, and the gastrointestinal (GI) tract secrete certain hormones.

There are different control mechanisms to stimulate or inhibit hormone secretions, including simple (negative or positive) feedback, complex feedback, nervous system control, and physiologic rhythms. Negative feedback, which works like a thermostat, is the most common means of control. Some hormones, such as cortisol, are released predictably with certain rhythms, such as the daily circadian rhythm.

Highlighted briefly here are a few major hormones released by the adrenal glands, pituitary, thyroid, parathyroid glands, and pancreas:

- The adrenal medulla (the inner part of the adrenal gland) secretes catecholamine hormones, such as epinephrine (adrenaline), norepinephrine, and dopamine. (When secreted by nerve cells, catecholamines are considered to be neurotransmitters.) Epinephrine and norepinephrine contribute to the "fight-or-flight" response induced by sympathetic nervous stimulation, which causes vasoconstriction and cardiac stimulation; stress or anger increases their release, thereby increasing blood pressure and heartbeat.
- The adrenal cortex (the outer part of the adrenal gland) secretes dozens of steroid hormones, including glucocorticoids such as cortisol (commercially available as

Hormones Released by the Adrenal Glands	Main Physiologic Effects
Catecholamines (from the medulla) Examples: epinephrine, norepinephrine, dopamine	Enhance sympathetic fight-or-flight stress responses; vasoconstriction; cardiac stimulation
Glucocorticoids (from the cortex) Example: hydrocortisone	Reduce inflammation; regulate metabolism and stress/immune responses
Mineralocorticoids (from the cortex) Example: aldosterone	Retain sodium and fluid; excrete potassium
Androgens (from the cortex) Example: testosterone	Enhance sex characteristics

hydrocortisone), mineralocorticoids such as aldosterone, and androgens such as testosterone. These hormones produce many different physiologic effects.

- The anterior pituitary gland releases several major hormones that regulate important body functions. Among them are growth hormone (GH), thyroid-stimulating hormone (TSH), and adrenocorticotropic hormone (ACTH); ACTH stimulates the adrenal glands to produce corticoid hormones.

- The posterior pituitary gland, which is essentially or anatomically an extension of the hypothalamus, secretes antidiuretic hormone (ADH) and oxytocin; both of these hormones are actually produced in the hypothalamus. ADH causes renal tubules to reabsorb water and reduce urine production. Oxytocin causes uterine smooth muscle to contract during labor, and milk to eject from the breast in lactating women.

- The thyroid gland releases thyroxine (T_4) and triiodothyronine (T_3), which primarily increase metabolism, thereby promoting growth, brain functions, and other neurologic activities. The secretion of thyroid hormones is dependent on the TSH level and iodine supply. The thyroid gland also releases calcitonin in response to a high blood calcium level; this hormone enhances the movement of calcium into the bones and the renal excretion of calcium. At a glance, the functions of these hormones are as follows:

Hormones Released by the Thyroid	Main Effects on Target Tissue
T_3 and T_4: production requires iodine; secretion stimulated by TSH	Increase metabolism and cellular growth; affect neurologic functions (T_4 is a precursor to T_3, which is a more potent hormone.)
Calcitonin: released when blood calcium level rises	Lowers blood calcium levels by moving calcium into the bones; not a critical factor in maintaining calcium balance

- The parathyroid glands secrete parathyroid hormone (PTH) to raise the blood calcium concentration when this level falls (in a negative feedback mechanism). PTH promotes bone resorption (bone breakdown, which releases the bone minerals, including calcium, into the blood) and inhibits bone formation. In addition, it stimulates the kidney's conversion of vitamin D to its most active form (1,25-dihydroxyvitamin D_3), which promotes the intestinal absorption of calcium.

Blood calcium level falls	PTH secretion increases to raise the calcium level by accelerating bone breakdown, which releases calcium into the blood; increasing D_3 level; promoting calcium absorption; and enhancing phosphate excretion
Blood calcium level rises	PTH secretion decreases

- The pancreas is both an exocrine and an endocrine gland. Its alpha cells secrete glucagon into the blood to increase the blood sugar level when needed; its beta cells release insulin, which facilitates glucose to move across the cell membranes into most of the cells for use, thereby lowering the blood sugar concentration.

Hormones Released by the Pancreas Gland	Functions
Glucagon: released when blood sugar is low; converts glycogen to glucose in the liver, thereby increasing blood sugar level	Increases blood glucose level
Insulin: released when blood sugar is high; helps glucose move into most of the cells	Decreases blood glucose level

Some cells in certain organs are not dependent on insulin for glucose use, such as cells in the brain, nerves, kidney tubules, and lens of the eye, among others.

DISORDERS AND CONDITIONS

ADDISON'S DISEASE/ADRENOCORTICAL INSUFFICIENCY

Primary Addison's disease, which involves adrenal hypofunction or insufficiency, originates within the gland itself. It is characterized by decreases in the secretion of glucocorticoids, mineralocorticoids, and androgen hormones.

In secondary adrenal hypofunction, glucocorticoid secretion is decreased, whereas aldosterone secretion often remains normal. The decreased glucocorticoid secretion may be related to low secretion of adrenocorticotropic hormone, steroid therapy interruption, or pituitary injury due to factors such as an autoimmune process or a tumor.

Adrenal (addisonian) crisis may arise from acute stress, such as trauma, infection, or interruption of steroid therapy; it causes a critical deficiency of mineralocorticoid and glucocorticoid hormones. If adrenal crisis is not treated, serious or fatal consequences may result.

Main Symptoms

In primary Addison's disease, patients are usually intolerant of strenuous activities and prone to infections or injuries because they do not have sufficient adrenal hormones to mount an adequate immune response or cope with stresses. The major symptoms of primary Addison's disease are as follows:

- Constant fatigue, muscle weakness, and stress intolerance
- Anorexia, weight loss, nausea, vomiting, and signs of dehydration
- Craving for salty foods due to low blood aldosterone levels, which frequently results in salt retention
- Abnormal skin coloration or suntanned appearance (due to release of melanocyte-stimulating hormone [MSH])

Secondary adrenal insufficiency may present with similar symptoms, but (1) without the characteristic hyperpigmentation, because the serum aldosterone level is often normal, so MSH release also remains normal, and (2) without affecting blood pressure or electrolyte balance.

In adrenal crisis, clinical features may include profound weakness, nausea and vomiting, and signs of circulatory shock with rapid pulse and respiration, apprehension, hypotension, and pallor or cyanosis.

Selected Nursing Tips

1. Therapy often includes treating underlying conditions, controlling blood pressure, correcting any electrolyte imbalances and hormone deficiencies, and preventing circulatory shock. Administer the prescribed steroid medicine with food to avoid gastric irritation.
2. Record daily weight and fluid intake and output. In primary Addison's disease, when patients have low aldosterone levels, slightly increasing sodium and fluid intake in times of stress, if indicated and appropriate, may prevent postural hypotension.
3. In case of physical stress, the physician should be notified to evaluate the patient with Addison's disease and possibly adjust or increase the dosage of steroid medication to prevent adrenal crisis—that is, a critical deficiency of glucocorticoids and mineralocorticoids.
4. Counsel patients about stress reduction measures and the necessity of carrying a medic alert card to alert medical personnel in case of emergencies.

Points to Consider

1. The benefits of steroid therapy must always be weighed against the serious risks of such treatment. Steroids may mask the signs of infection and have immunosuppressive or other serious side effects, including inducing diabetes, peptic ulceration, glaucoma, cataract, or osteoporosis.

Long-term therapy with corticosteroids can also induce Cushing's syndrome, which causes changes in multiple body systems.

2. Be aware of the increased risk of adrenal insufficiency in any patient who has been undergoing steroid medication therapy. Abrupt cessation of steroid therapy may cause fatal circulatory collapse.

3. When serum aldosterone level is low (as in primary Addison's disease), the kidneys will excrete more sodium and less potassium, leading to a low serum sodium level (and, in turn, low blood volume and pressure) and a higher potassium level. Unless treated promptly, hyperkalemia could lead to dysrhythmia or cardiac arrest. After steroid replacement, assess for signs of hypokalemia, which may result from the presence of excessive mineralocorticoids.

4. Maintenance doses of steroid medicine should be taken exactly as prescribed.

5. Adrenal (addisonian) crisis may occur with trauma, physiologic stress, or failure to take steroid medications in patients with chronic adrenal insufficiency. It is a medical emergency, requiring immediate effective treatment.

Precautions

1. Steroid tablets should not be crushed, dissolved, or broken during administration, so as to prevent an abrupt increase in the drug level and to maintain the drug's therapeutic effects.

2. Monitor serum electrolytes and bone density test results in patients with adrenal conditions; be alert for signs of infection. Assess the oral cavity for signs of yeast infection, such as white patches on the tongue, a side effect of steroids.

CUSHING'S SYNDROME

Cushing's syndrome—a constellation of clinical abnormalities involving several different body systems—usually results from excessive amounts of corticosteroids in the blood, especially glucocorticoids. Possible factors inducing this condition include long-term use of glucocorticoid medication (e.g., prednisone), overproduction of ACTH due to a pituitary tumor, and other mechanisms.

Long-term use of corticosteroids, even at therapeutic doses, can have serious complications. Excessive levels of corticosteroids can disturb serum glucose and electrolyte balance. The patient may develop insulin resistance, exhibiting signs of diabetes mellitus.

Mineralocorticoid aldosterone excess, though relatively rare, can cause the kidneys to excrete potassium and retain sodium, thereby increasing fluid volume and contributing to hypertension or heart failure.

Main Symptoms

- Behavior and body image changes with typical trunk obesity; fat pads over the upper back or on the face and thin extremities
- Sodium and fluid retention, hypertension, and hyperglycemia
- Peptic (mostly gastric) ulcers
- Hypokalemia, and muscle wasting and weakness

Selected Nursing Tips

1. The primary goal of management of Cushing's syndrome is to restore hormone balance and reverse any underlying disease process. Treatment may depend on the root cause and underlying condition; possible therapeutic modalities include radiation, surgery, drugs, and other approaches.
2. In patients with Cushing's syndrome, monitor vital signs and lab results for hypertension, hypernatremia, hypokalemia, hyperglycemia, and glycosuria (glucose in urine).
   Advise patients to decrease their carbohydrate and salt intake, while increasing protein and potassium intake as indicated.
3. When patients are on long-term corticosteroid therapy after removal of the bilateral adrenal glands or the pituitary

gland (often due to hormone-producing pathology of the glands), emphasize the importance of taking hormone replacement medication exactly as prescribed and the need to seek medical attention if symptoms of possible inadequate dose or overdose occur, especially when the patient is receiving mineralocorticoid therapy. Inadequate-dose symptoms may include weakness, postural hypotension, and dizziness, while overdose symptoms may include severe swelling and weight gain. Monitor for signs of adverse effects, including insomnia, mood swings, increased susceptibility to infection, and delayed wound healing.

Points to Consider

1. Patients should be assured that most of the physical changes due to Cushing's syndrome can be managed with proper treatment.
2. Long-term steroid therapy can predispose patients to osteoporosis, resulting from the movement of minerals out of the bones and decreased bone density. Osteoporosis may cause pathologic fractures, which necessitate implementation of extra precautions.

Precaution

Interruption or abrupt discontinuation of corticosteroid therapy can lead to fatal adrenal insufficiency. Steroid medications must be gradually tapered off as ordered when cessation of therapy is deemed necessary.

DIABETES INSIPIDUS

Diabetes insipidus (DI) often results from an antidiuretic hormone (ADH) insufficiency or the kidney's unresponsiveness to ADH, leading to excretion of water (without water being reabsorbed). Thus, clinical findings in DI include increased thirst and urine output.

This form of diabetes may be transient or chronic, stemming from diverse pathologies, including tumors, head trauma, and infections, or occurring with use of certain drugs. The specific cause of DI is unclear.

Main Symptoms

The onset of DI may be abrupt, with its major features including the following:

- Nearly colorless urine, polyuria (excessive urination), and low urine specific gravity (more dilute)
- Polydipsia (excessive thirst)
- Signs of dehydration (poor skin turgor, dry mucous membranes, hypotension, irritability, dizziness, and constipation) and weight loss
- High serum sodium level (hypernatremia) and osmolality due to pure water loss

Selected Nursing Tips

1. Nursing care includes ensuring easy access to drinking water or adequate fluid replacement to prevent dehydration and adhering to the dosing schedule for therapies. Monitor the patient's urine output, daily weight, and serum sodium level.
2. Obtain baseline vital signs, weight, serum electrolytes, and urine specific gravity. Patients with DI may have large amounts of almost colorless urine with low specific-gravity values (and an elevated serum sodium level), and may experience significant weight loss.
3. Educate patients to recognize the signs of inadequate medication, as reflected by urine output exceeding fluid intake and recurrence of polyuria.

Points to Consider

1. A fluid-deprivation test may be ordered to help determine the underlying cause of the patient's DI. The patient undergoing the test should be monitored closely, including frequent checks of vital signs, urine output, and weight, to be compared with the baseline data. If a significant change

in the vital signs or weight is noted, the test should be discontinued and the patient treated immediately with fluid replacement or medication.

2. Desmopressin (DDAVP), a synthetic form of vasopressin hormone that has antidiuretic effects, is often used to treat diabetes insipidus. It promotes water reabsorption by increasing the permeability of the renal collecting ducts and decreasing urine output. Signs of water intoxication (dilutional hyponatremia)—a potential side effect of excessive doses of desmopressin—may include headache, drowsiness, confusion, reduced urination, rapid weight gain, and seizures.

3. DI resulting from certain causes, such as head trauma, is often self-limiting; it improves when the underlying condition is treated and improved.

Precautions

1. Monitor for signs of hypovolemic shock by assessing vital signs closely, especially during a water deprivation test.

2. Follow the guidelines for proper fluid replacement to avoid over-hydration.

DIABETES MELLITUS

Diabetes mellitus (DM) is characterized by chronic metabolic disturbances of glucose, protein, and fat. It often results from insulin deficiency, insulin resistance, or both.

Diabetes is derived from a Greek word meaning "to siphon," referring to the excessive urination associated with DM. *Mellitus* originates from a Latin word meaning "sweet."

In type 1 DM, the pancreatic beta cells are destroyed or their functions are reduced, resulting in absent or insufficient insulin production. Genetic predisposition, immunologic beta-cell destruction, and environmental influences (e.g., viral exposure) are thought to be contributing factors to the development of this form of DM. The onset is often rapid and acute. In contrast to type 2 diabetes, there are usually no complications at diagnosis.

In type 2 DM, which is much more prevalent than type 1 DM, the tissues are not able to use insulin effectively, either because of insufficient insulin production or because of the tissues' resistance to insulin. Its manifestations may appear so gradually that a patient often attributes the nonspecific symptoms, such as fatigue and recurrent infection, to other problems, leading to a missed diagnosis until serious complications occur. Overweight patients tend to develop insulin resistance due to insufficient or unresponsive insulin receptors. In patients with insulin resistance or insufficiency, oral antidiabetic medication helps release the insulin that the body has produced.

	Type 1 DM	Type 2 DM
Onset of disease	Rapid and acute onset	Slow onset, undiagnosed for years with symptoms mimicking those of other problems
Insulin production	Minimal or absent production of insulin	Diminished insulin utilization and secretion over time
Signs and symptoms	Hyperglycemia (high blood sugar/ glucose level; polyuria (excessive urination); polydipsia (excessive thirst); polyphagia (excessive eating); weight loss, fatigue, thin frame	Nonspecific; may have hyperglycemia, polyuria, polydipsia infections, vision changes, fatigue, and delayed wound healing; often overweight (with no weight loss or polyphagia)
Usual treatments	Insulin injections, planned diet, and exercise	Oral agents or/and insulin injections, planned diet, exercise
Complications	Often none at diagnosis; possibly diabetic ketoacidosis (DKA) and others	May have at diagnosis; possibly hyperglycemic-hyperosmolar state (HHS), and others

Main Symptoms

In type 1 DM, the initial characteristic symptoms are often acute with a rapid onset. Patients may exhibit polydipsia, polyuria, and polyphagia; these symptoms result from hyperglycemia, due to a lack of insulin to transfer glucose into the cells to be used as energy.

Patients with type 2 DM may also experience hyperglycemia, though it is often not as severe as that seen in type 1 DM, with accompanying symptoms such as polyuria or polydipsia. They may also have blurred vision, fatigue, skin problems, or delayed wound healing resulting from hyperglycemia. Polyphagia and weight loss are not common in patients with type 2 DM.

Hyperglycemia causes an increased serum osmotic pressure, pulling fluids out of body tissues, leading to osmotic diuresis, polyuria, excessive thirst, dry mucous membranes, and poor skin turgor.

When the circulating glucose level exceeds the renal threshold for absorbing this molecule, the excess glucose will spill into the urine; thus urinalysis will be positive for glucose in the urine (**glycosuria**). The patient will also experience symptoms of weight loss, hunger, and fatigue as sugar is wasted in the urine.

An excess of insulin in the blood can lead to low blood sugar (hypoglycemia). Hypoglycemia can directly affect the patient's mental status because the brain needs a constant supply

Symptoms of Hyperglycemia	Symptoms of Hypoglycemia
Elevated blood sugar, increased urination, glycosuria, increased appetite and thirst, fatigue, weakness, abdominal cramps, nausea and vomiting, blurred vision, potential DKA (mostly in type 1 DM) or HHS (in type 2 DM)	Low blood sugar, cold/clammy skin, rapid pulse, hunger, nervousness, tremor; decreased alertness, dizziness, emotional change, confusion, slurred speech, potential seizures or coma

of sufficient glucose to function normally. Low blood sugar can also stimulate the release of epinephrine (adrenaline), which in turn can cause vasoconstriction and trigger symptoms ranging from tremor, tachycardia, cold sweat, and irrational behavior to loss of consciousness.

Selected Nursing Tips

1. Nursing management aims at controlling the blood glucose level and preventing complications. Check the patient's glucose level regularly and when signs of hypoglycemia are noted.

2. In a conscious patient with hypoglycemia, a simple sugar, such as a glass of orange juice or prescribed oral glucagon gel, may reverse the symptoms. Glucagon injection may be indicated (often per standing order) for a patient who becomes unable to drink due to hypoglycemia. Giving food containing carbohydrates and protein later may produce sustained effects.

3. If the body has not produced insulin that can be released, oral antidiabetic medication will not have any effect. In such case, the glucose level is mainly controlled by insulin injections in conjunction with other measures.

4. While administering insulin, it is important to rotate the injection sites so as to prevent insulin lipodystrophy (altered fat tissue at the injection site), which can affect normal insulin absorption.

5. The abdomen is a preferred site for insulin injection, because absorption is more even and rapid in this site than when insulin is injected in the extremities.

6. Make sure the patient is able to demonstrate (after being taught) the correct techniques of insulin administration.

7. Type 2 DM is commonly managed through diet, exercise, and oral antidiabetic medications. Encourage patients to exercise regularly, as this kind of physical activity can lower blood glucose level by increasing tissue sensitivity to insulin and

increasing the number of insulin receptors. Weight reduction in some patients can also decrease insulin resistance.

8. Hypoglycemia may occur in response to strenuous exercise. Advise patients to avoid exercising at the peak time of the insulin they have administered. The result of a capillary glucose (finger stick) test before exercise may be used to decide whether or how much of a snack is needed.

9. Tailor education to the needs and abilities of patients with diabetes; teach them to identify signs of hypoglycemia and hyperglycemia so as to get prompt treatment. Monitor for signs of the development of complications, including diabetic neuropathy or nephropathy (e.g., end-stage kidney disease), retinopathy (e.g., gradual loss of vision), and cardiovascular impairment.

Points to Consider

1. Insulin is the main regulator of the metabolism and storage of ingested carbohydrates, fats, and protein. Insulin enables glucose to enter the cells to be used for energy or deposited as glycogen in the liver and muscle cells, with a few exceptions; cells not dependent on insulin for glucose absorption include the cells of the brain, nerves, and intestinal mucosa, among others.

   - Without insulin, glucose cannot enter insulin-dependent cells to be utilized or converted to glycogen for storage. Glucose remaining in the blood causes the blood sugar level to climb.

   - The blood potassium level can be affected by insulin production or administration because insulin promotes potassium transport into the cells (i.e., potassium accompanies glucose into the cells). The serum potassium level may decrease as a result of excessive insulin administration, potentially leading to dangerous hypokalemia.

2. Glucagon produced in the pancreatic alpha cells has the opposite effect of insulin. It converts glycogen to glucose in

the liver, and complements other mechanisms that increase blood sugar in time of need. Prescribed glucagon is available in oral and injection preparations to treat hypoglycemia. When hypoglycemic patients are not able to ingest anything orally due to decreased alertness, glucagon injection may be indicated as ordered.

3. Hemoglobin A_{1c} is a minor component of hemoglobin that most strongly combines with glucose. The Hb A_{1c} test measures the amount of glucose attached to hemoglobin over approximately a 3-month period, which is the life span of red blood cells. It provides a long-term index of the individual's average blood glucose level.

   - The test result reflects an average blood glucose level, or how well glucose has been controlled over the past few months.
   - Urine tests for glucose and ketones indicate blood glucose control over only the previous few hours.

4. The dawn phenomenon and the Somogyi phenomenon both refer to high fasting blood sugar in the morning, but the causative mechanisms are different. Identifying the pattern and trend of glucose levels over time may help patients manage their diabetes. Knowing the possible causes of hyperglycemia may suggest approaches to prevent its occurrence in some patients.

   - The dawn phenomenon refers to hyperglycemia in the morning before eating, possibly due to the secretion of growth and steroid hormones before dawn. Blood glucose levels may rise in patients with diabetes because their insulin production is inadequate.
   - The Somogyi phenomenon is a high fasting blood glucose level after an undetected episode of hypoglycemia during sleep. The release of counter-regulatory hormones, such as growth or steroid hormones, is thought to cause this rebound hyperglycemia. Patients may complain of symptoms such as night sweats. Blood sugar (BS) can be checked between approximately 2 AM and

4 AM to confirm hypoglycemic status so that proper preventive measures can be identified and adopted.

Types of High Fasting Glucose Levels in the Morning

	Dawn Phenomenon	Somogyi Phenomenon (Rebound Hyperglycemia)
Causative mechanisms	Predawn normal release of hormones (e.g., growth hormone or cortisol) causing hyperglycemia in individuals with inadequate insulin	Extra hormones released due to early-morning undetected hypoglycemia leading to rebound hyperglycemia
Therapeutic approaches	Better timing of insulin administration	Check blood sugar level—add snack or adjust dosage as ordered

5. Complications associated with DM may involve multiple systems with different presentations, including renal, neurologic, or cardiovascular abnormalities. Nurses can play an important role in educating patients about the importance of controlling blood glucose levels and thereby reducing the risk of developing serious complications. A few of these complications are discussed next.
   - Hyperglycemic-hyperosmolar state (HHS) is a serious complication of type 2 DM. Patients are usually dehydrated and have severe hyperglycemia. Manifestations of HHS may range from sensory-motor impairment to coma. A life-threatening syndrome, HHS differs from diabetic ketoacidosis in that there is an absence of, or minimal level of, ketone bodies in either the blood or the urine. Patients with HHS still have enough circulating

insulin to prevent ketoacidosis, but not enough to transport glucose to the cells and prevent hyperglycemia and
its subsequent results. When HHS is suspected, closely
monitor the patient's cardiac, renal, and mental status
and participate in collaborative care. Nursing management includes reducing the blood glucose level, correcting fluid and electrolyte imbalances, eliminating the
precipitating cause, and preventing complications.

- Diabetes ketoacidosis (DKA) is a state of metabolic acidosis, characterized by hyperglycemia, ketosis, acidosis,
and dehydration. It results from profound insulin deficiency, often occurring in patients with type 1 DM.
  - Patients may have ketonuria. When not enough insulin is available to transfer glucose into the cells for
  use as energy, fat or protein is broken down for energy; acidic ketones are formed as by-products of this
  process.
  - Frequent urination (resulting from hyperglycemia and
  osmotic diuresis) can lead to loss of fluid and electrolytes. Dehydration and hypovolemia (low blood volume) can affect cardiac and renal functions.
  - Patients may present with Kussmaul's respirations
  (deep/gasping breathing) as the lungs attempt to compensate for the lowered pH by blowing off (exhaling) CO_2. Fruity breath odor and change of level of
  consciousness may be found in patients with diabetic
  ketoacidosis. Follow the nursing care guidelines; be
  aware that potassium will enter the cells with insulin
  when therapy starts to correct hyperglycemia and hy-
  perketonemia, potentially resulting in hypokalemia.
  (Potassium replacement must be carefully administered to prevent hyperkalemia, which can also lead to
  cardiac arrhythmia or arrest.)
  - Therapy for DKA may include reducing the blood
  glucose level, restoring fluid volume, managing electrolyte imbalances, and reversing acidosis. Monitor

for signs of hypoglycemia in patients receiving regular insulin for hyperglycemia.

- ◆ An improved condition may be evidenced by the patient's becoming alert and oriented and having good skin turgor. Patients' blood glucose levels should be monitored frequently to prevent recurrence of DKA.
- ■ Foot complications may result from injuries to the lower extremities. Patients with either type of DM may have some degree of peripheral neuropathy and loss of protective sensation, which places them at higher risk for injury to their feet. Teach patients to:
  - ◆ Carefully examine their feet every day, even using a mirror if necessary, and take every means to prevent ulceration.
  - ◆ Treat injuries promptly, particularly those on the lower extremities.
  - ◆ Wear socks and well-fitting shoes because they may not feel pain in the feet.

Precaution

Meticulous blood glucose control is essential to prevent serious complications of DM, such as blindness, myocardial infarction, stroke, and end-stage renal disease. Hypoglycemia must be treated immediately. Advise patients to follow treatment regimens, including observing sick-day guidelines—that is, carefully managing their blood glucose level when they have minor illness.

PARATHYROID DISORDERS

The parathyroid glands release PTH or parathormone with a negative feedback mechanism based on blood calcium levels: their secretion of the hormone increases when blood calcium decreases, and decreases when blood calcium increases.

The secretion of PTH can also be influenced by other factors, such as the level of active vitamin D, which may affect GI absorption of calcium and the blood calcium level.

(Calcitonin, in contrast to PTH, moves calcium into the bones, thereby reducing the serum calcium level.)

Hyperparathyroidism

Hyperparathyroidism is characterized by overproduction of PTH or parathormone. Excessive PTH concentrations can increase blood calcium level by enhancing calcium absorption and promoting bone decalcification. High serum calcium levels increase the risk that calcium-containing stones will form in the kidney.

Overproduction of PTH may have several different etiologies. For example, it may be due to parathyroid enlargement or occur secondary to a condition that causes hypocalcemia, such as vitamin D deficiency, and a subsequent excessive compensatory response.

Main Symptoms

The manifestations of hyperparathyroidism usually result from hypercalcemia, reflecting abnormalities in various systems:

- Renal calculi (stones) and polyuria due to increased serum osmotic pressure
- Osteopenia (decreased bone density) and greater susceptibility to fracture
- Nausea, vomiting, and constipation
- Mood disorder, personality disturbance, and stupor
- Muscle weakness, lower back pain, and cardiac arrhythmias

Serious complications may include renal failure or pancreatic and other abnormalities.

Selected Nursing Tips

1. Treatment varies depending on the etiology, but often focuses on eliminating the source of hyperparathyroidism or the root causes of parathyroid hyperplasia. Various therapies may be used to decrease calcium levels and prevent complications resulting from the disorder or its treatment.

2. Increased fluid intake may decrease the likelihood of stone formation, often with calcium as a component. It is believed that cranberry juice may increase urine acidity and reduce urinary pH.

3. Restricting dietary calcium intake and avoiding calcium-containing antacids may be indicated when the root cause is not removed; administer prescribed medications to promote excretion of calcium to lower its serum level.

4. Encourage ambulation as appropriate to prevent formation of kidney stones; the patient's urine may need to be screened for possible presence of calculi.

5. Protect the patient from injuries by taking safety measures to prevent pathologic fractures; keep the bed at a low position and handle the patient gently to minimize stress on the bones.

Points to Consider

1. Monitor and compare laboratory results to detect trends; report signs of problems promptly. To reverse hypercalcemic crisis and prevent potentially life-threatening neurologic, cardiovascular, and renal complications, specialists' assessment and care of the patient are essential.

2. Surgical therapy may be indicated to remove the source of PTH overproduction. Provide postoperative care per nursing guidelines and the facility's protocol. After parathyroidectomy, position the patient as required with head and neck properly supported, and monitor for signs of respiratory distress and complications, such as laryngeal nerve damage, hemorrhage, and swelling at the incision site.

Precaution

After parathyroidectomy, keep emergency supplies and medications readily available (e.g., calcium gluconate for acute hypocalcemia). Patients may have tingling sensation in the hands and around the mouth, which usually subsides shortly after the surgery; however, this sensation can also be an early sign of severe tetany or hypocalcemia. Monitor the patient closely.

Hypoparathyroidism

Hypoparathyroidism, an insufficiency of PTH, can have a variety of etiologies, including injury or accidental removal of the parathyroid glands during thyroid or other neck surgery. A low serum PTH level and hypocalcemia may lead to tetany or spasmodic contractions.

Main Symptoms

Hypoparathyroidism presents with clinical features of low blood calcium (and high phosphatemia), including the following signs and symptoms:

- Positive Chvostek's sign (facial spasm when tapped)
- Neuromuscular irritability, muscle cramps, or tingling sensations
- (Acute) tetany, which may cause laryngospasm, stridor, cyanosis, or seizure, possibly starting with a tingling in the hands or around the mouth

Selected Nursing Tips

1. Monitor patients with hypoparathyroidism for signs of tetany with tingling sensation; watch for signs of laryngospasm, such as respiratory stridor or difficulty swallowing (dysphagia).
2. Calcium-rich foods, such as dairy and soy products and green leafy vegetables, may be recommended as part of the patient's diet. Food high in vitamin D may increase GI absorption of calcium.
3. Calcium (e.g., calcium gluconate) must be infused slowly at the prescribed rate to prevent hypotension and bradycardia; rapid administration may cause vasodilation and its serious consequences, including arrhythmias or cardiac arrest.

Point to Consider

For patients with chronic hypoparathyroidism, a high-calcium, low-phosphate diet may be prescribed. Some foods such as egg yolk, though high in calcium, may not be recommended due to their high phosphorus content. Spinach contains oxalate, which may contribute to the formation of insoluble calcium compounds.

Precaution

Monitor a patient who has had a thyroid gland removal (thyroidectomy) or neck surgery for signs of tetany; a worrisome sign is a low serum calcium level with tingling sensation due to possibly accidental parathyroid gland removal owing to the proximity of the parathyroid glands to the thyroid. Have emergency equipment in a designated place for easy access, such as IV calcium preparations, a tracheotomy tray, or an endotracheal tube.

PHEOCHROMOCYTOMA

In pheochromocytoma, there is a tumor (often benign) of the adrenal medulla that leads to production of excessive amounts of epinephrine and norepinephrine (catecholamines). The sympathetic nervous system may be activated, evidenced by hypertension accompanied by headache, diaphoresis, and palpitation. If untreated, pheochromocytoma is potentially fatal.

Main Symptoms

The excessive secretion of one or more catecholamine hormones, such as epinephrine or norepinephrine, can cause the classic presentation of pheochromocytoma:

- Hypertension, persistent or episodic
- Headache, tremor, and nervousness
- Hyperglycemia
- Heartbeat increase (tachycardia), palpitation, dyspnea, and vertigo
- Sweating (diaphoresis), pallor, and warmth
- Polyuria, nausea, vomiting, and abdominal pain

Selected Nursing Tips

1. Manage an acute hypertensive crisis by administering medication to normalize blood pressure. Remind patients

on antihypertensives, such as propranolol (Inderal), to get up slowly so as to prevent postural hypotension, and not to stop the medication abruptly or take over-the-counter cold medications (stimulants) without their physician's approval.

2. Check blood pressure as often as indicated to detect transient or episodic blood pressure spikes, and to help monitor the effectiveness of therapy.

3. Schedule care to allow needed undisturbed rest. Ensure a quiet, cool environment because this condition may cause profuse sweating. Maintain the patient's nutritional status.

4. Nurses may assist in pheochromocytoma case finding; when patients do not respond to conventional hypertension treatments, but have episodic headache, palpitations, and sweating, suspicion for this condition may be raised. Ensure the reliability of urine catecholamine measurements to help establish the diagnosis.

Point to Consider

Before initiating 24-hour urine collection, remind the patient to avoid certain medications and foods high in vanillin as per the lab's requirements (e.g., chocolate, banana, caffeine).

Precaution

Check blood pressure frequently or every few minutes, as indicated, especially after surgery or administering potent medications. Drastic fluctuations in blood pressure often occur after adrenal-gland manipulation or surgery. Corticosteroids replacement may become necessary in some patients.

SYNDROME OF INAPPROPRIATE ANTIDIURETIC HORMONE

In syndrome of inappropriate antidiuretic hormone (SIADH) secretion, there is an overproduction of antidiuretic hormone.

SIADH often results from a malignancy, such as small cell lung cancer, which can produce, store, or release ADH regardless of its serum osmolality. SIADH secondary to head injury or certain medications tends to be self-limiting.

Main Symptoms

- Inability to urinate, oliguria (diminished urine), and weight gain despite anorexia or vomiting
- Muscle cramping or twitching—an early sign of sodium imbalance
- Dilutional hyponatremia (low serum sodium level/water intoxication) and fluid retention (due to excessive secretion of ADH)

Neurologic symptoms may develop rapidly when the serum sodium level continues to fall. Severe hyponatremia may potentially result in cerebral edema; that is, the decreased serum osmolality causes fluid to move into the brain cells. Personality changes, lethargy, seizures, or coma may ensue.

Edema is not evident because fluid is widely distributed in different compartments of the body.

Selected Nursing Tips

1. Correct the underlying cause when possible.
2. With severe hyponatremia, fluid restriction may be ordered to relieve the symptoms and prevent water intoxication. Provide a hazard-free and quiet environment; implement seizure precautions.
3. Monitor the patient's weight, level of consciousness, urine output, and serum osmolality to determine his or her fluid volume status.

Point to Consider

The major differences between DI and SIADH are summarized here for quick reference.

	DI	SIADH
ADH level	Low	High
Urine output	Excess	Scarce; unable to excrete a dilute urine
Possible causes	Problems with ADH-producing glands or other disorders, head injury, certain drugs	Malignancy, other conditions, head injuries, certain drugs
Some major symptoms	Increased thirst and urination, hypernatremia; weight loss, low urine specific gravity/colorless urine	Dilutional hyponatremia; weight gain, muscle weakness, potential cerebral edema

Desired outcomes of SIADH treatment can be evidenced by increased urine output and weight reduction.

Precaution

If hypertonic saline is prescribed for a patient with severe hyponatremia, an infusion pump is required to ensure a very slow infusion rate (as ordered) to prevent a rapid increase in plasma sodium. Monitor for signs of fluid overload (e.g., crackles in the lungs, bounding pulse, peripheral edema), which may potentially lead to pulmonary edema, a life-threatening complication.

THYROID DISORDERS

The thyroid gland secretes both thyroxine (T_4) and triiodothyronine (T_3)—hormones that help regulate cellular metabolism and promote normal growth, thereby influencing all major body systems. Iodine is needed in the production of thyroid hormone. Both hyperthyroidism and hypothyroidism are common endocrine disorders.

Hyperthyroidism

In hyperthyroidism, thyroid gland hyperactivity results in an increased release of thyroid hormone (TH). This condition may be traced to various causes or precipitators, including genetic or autoimmune factors, high serum TSH levels, too much thyroid medication, or excessive intake of iodine.

Thyrotoxicosis (physiologic manifestations of hyperthyroidism) can be precipitated by serious physical or emotional stress. Thyroid storm is a rare, life-threatening condition of hyperthyroidism, in which symptoms of hyperthyroidism are more acute and often fatal, requiring immediate vigorous treatment.

Main Symptoms

The assessment findings for hyperthyroidism are usually associated with increased metabolism and signs of an activated sympathetic nervous system, resulting from excessive thyroid hormones:

- Nervousness, insomnia, and heat intolerance
- Palpitation, tremor, and increased sweating
- Weight loss despite increased appetite, plus nutritional deficits
- Exophthalmos (bulging eyeballs), which is often seen in some patients with Graves' disease, a common form of hyperthyroidism

Elderly patients with hyperthyroidism may exhibit vague or nonspecific symptoms.

Goiter—an enlargement of the thyroid gland—can be related to any condition that leads to hyperfunction or hypofunction of the gland, including hyperthyroidism or hypothyroidism, other thyroid problems, and a lack of iodine in the diet.

Symptoms of thyroid storm may range from agitation, hypertension, rapid heartbeat, fever, and delirium to coma.

Selected Nursing Tips

1. The treatment of hyperthyroidism is largely aimed at reducing the excessive thyroid hormone production, relieving

symptoms, and preventing complications; therapies may include drugs, surgery, or radioactive iodine. Radioactive iodine therapy reduces thyroid hormone secretion by damaging or destroying the thyroid gland, but its main side effect is hypothyroidism.

2. Antithyroid medication must be taken exactly as prescribed; monitor the patient's pulse and weight daily.

3. Patients with hyperthyroidism need a high-calorie, high-protein diet to meet the body's energy demands and prevent weight loss. A restful environment is more conducive to recovery.

4. The patient with exophthalmos may prefer to use tinted glasses. If patients cannot close their eyes, eyelids may be taped shut while they sleep, if recommended by their physician, so as to prevent serious corneal injury.

Points to Consider

Following a thyroidectomy, provide nursing care per guidelines. Postoperative care may include the following measures:

- Assess the patient for signs of possible laryngeal nerve damage (e.g., asking the patient a simple question at regular intervals and listening for the quality of the patient's voice); postoperative hoarseness is usually temporary.
- Watch for signs of tetany due to hypocalcemia resulting from an accidental removal of the parathyroid gland during a thyroid surgery. IV calcium preparations and other emergency equipment and supplies should be readily available.
- Assess for signs of bleeding by checking the dressing on the side and back of the neck.
- Instruct the patient to support the head when coughing or changing positions.

Precaution

Thyroid crisis (storm), a serious complication, may occur in patients with hyperthyroidism, especially when they are under major stress. Avoid palpating the thyroid excessively to avoid precipitating thyroid storm. Its symptoms include elevated temperature, pulse, and blood pressure, plus increased irritability. Immediate intervention to stabilize the patient's hemodynamic status is indicated.

Hypothyroidism

Hypothyroidism—a state of insufficient serum thyroid hormones due to hypofunction of the thyroid gland—results in a lowered basal metabolism, affecting all body systems. It can stem from several abnormal conditions:

- Autoimmune thyroiditis (Hashimoto's disease) or inflammation
- A deficiency of thyroid-stimulating hormone (TSH)
- Treatments for hyperthyroidism, including thyroid surgery, radioactive iodine therapy, and antithyroid medications such as propylthiouracil (Propyl-Thyracil)
- Dietary iodine deficiency

Main Symptoms

The clinical characteristics of hypothyroidism are signs of slow metabolic rate:

- Fatigue or lethargy
- Impaired memory or slowed speech
- Constipation due to decreased GI motility
- Weight gain resulting from decreased metabolism
- Cardiac complications such as bradycardia (slow heart rate), which may be late signs

In older adults, hypothyroidism may have different manifestations.

Myxedema coma, a life-threatening complication, can be set off by major stresses in some patients with hypothyroidism, including trauma, infection, hypoglycemia, or hypoventilation due to the use of narcotics or withdrawal of thyroid medication.

The clinical features of myxedema coma may include the following:

- A puffy face, periorbital edema, or mask-like affect (apathy)
- Lower-than-normal temperature (hypothermia)
- Low blood pressure (hypotension)
- Low blood sugar (hypoglycemia)
- Depressed respiratory drive resulting in carbon dioxide retention and decreased level of consciousness, potentially progressing to coma

Selected Nursing Tips

1. Advise patients to consume a diet high in bulk and low in calories. Administer stool softeners or laxatives as needed per order.
2. Levothyroxine (Synthroid) is used for hypothyroidism and should be taken in the morning to coincide with normal hormone release. Taking the medication on an empty stomach 30 minutes before a meal can facilitate its absorption. Changing brands may cause problems with bioequivalence, resulting in less predictable patient responses.
3. Educate the patient to take thyroid medication as ordered (even if symptoms have subsided) to prevent myxedema.
4. Nursing management for myxedema coma includes maintaining vital functions and optimal oxygenation. Administer fluids cautiously as indicated to prevent water intoxication; monitor vital signs and watch for side effects of the medication administered to correct hypothyroidism.
5. In patients with underlying heart disease, thyroid hormone replacement may increase the workload on the heart and myocardial oxygen requirements; instruct patients to report cardiovascular problems, such as angina or reduced urine output, a possible sign of decreasing cardiac output.

Points to Consider

1. When hypothyroidism is suspected, evaluation of serum TSH, T_4, and T_3 levels is usually indicated.
2. Provide warm blankets or extra clothing to compensate for low body temperature. Note that rapid rewarming of a patient with hypothermia may cause vasodilation and potential vascular collapse.

Precaution

Medications must be taken as ordered. Thyroid hormone replacement can cause hyperthyroidism; watch for signs of restlessness, sweating, weight loss, difficulty sleeping, and having more bowel movements than are normal for the patient. Report such problems promptly as indicated; notify the prescriber of significant alterations in the patient's sleep and bowel-elimination patterns, which may help gauge the effectiveness of the hormone therapy and the need for dosage adjustment.

CHAPTER 7

Digestive Issues

The digestive system is primarily responsible for supplying nutrients to the body cells through ingestion, digestion, absorption, and elimination processes. It consists of the gastrointestinal (GI) tract and its accessory organs and glands. The tube-like GI tract includes the mouth, pharynx, esophagus, stomach, small intestine, large intestine, rectum, and anus.

The small intestine consists of three sections:

- The duodenum, the most proximal section
- The jejunum, the middle section
- The ileum, the distal section, which ends at the ileocecal orifice, the opening to the large intestine

The vermiform appendix is attached to the cecum, which forms the first portion of the large intestine. The large intestine consists of three sections located in the abdomen:

- The ascending colon, on the right
- The transverse colon, crossing the top from left to right
- The descending colon, on the left

The sigmoid colon, rectum, and anus constitute the last portion of the large intestine.

Absorption of nutrients and fluids, including vitamins and most electrolytes, primarily takes place in the small intestine.

The small intestine's absorption surface is greatly expanded by the structural presence of numerous villi, microvilli, and circular folds. A patient who has undergone a small intestine resection will have a decreased area for nutrient absorption—a factor that often results in vitamin deficiencies.

The associated digestive organs include the liver, pancreas, and gallbladder. The pancreas secretes a variety of digestive enzymes, including trypsin, amylase, and lipase, which aid in digesting protein, starch, and fats, respectively. Bile is secreted by the liver and stored in the gallbladder. When fatty food enters the duodenum, the gallbladder is stimulated to discharge bile into the common bile duct; from there, the bile enters the duodenum and aids in the digestion of fats.

Psychological and emotional factors, such as stress, cigarette smoking, and fatigue, can also affect GI function.

DISORDERS AND CONDITIONS

APPENDICITIS

Appendicitis involves an infection or inflammation of the appendix (a tube-like pouch attached to the cecum), often resulting from obstruction of its small lumen. Hardened fecal matter is frequently the culprit. Appendicitis can also be caused by a foreign body, parasites, inflammation, or other conditions that lead to obstruction and subsequent distension of the appendix with accumulation of mucus, bacteria, and pus. If untreated, a serious complication such as abscess or perforation may ensue.

Main Symptoms

- Abdominal cramping; constant pain, which eventually becomes localized (at McBurney's point) in the right lower quadrant of the abdomen; and rebound tenderness
- Fever

- Anorexia, vomiting, decreased bowel sounds, and abdominal rigidity

Elderly patients may have no symptoms or only vague discomfort, such as mild abdominal tenderness, until the appendix ruptures. The possible delay in seeking treatment increases the incidence of complications, such as appendix perforation, in that population.

Selected Nursing Tips

1. Nursing care may include relieving pain, maintaining fluid and electrolyte balance, eliminating infection, and preventing complications. Take measures to ward off dehydration and promote renal function; administer antibiotics or IV fluids as ordered.
2. In acute appendicitis, the patient should be placed on NPO (nil per os, meaning "nothing by mouth") status, to keep the stomach empty in anticipation of possible surgery.
3. Surgery is likely to be performed laparoscopically; follow the surgeon's instructions or facility's protocol for postoperative nursing care.
4. Monitor the patient's vital signs and intake/output; watch for signs or symptoms of peritonitis, such as abdominal distension, rigidity, and pain with increased pulse and respiration, which may result from appendix perforation, a serious complication.
5. After appendectomy, coughing, turning, deep breathing, and early ambulation by the patient may prevent pulmonary complications.

Points to Consider

1. Avoid palpating the abdomen of a patient with suspected appendicitis; ask the patient to cough to elicit the pain response. Sudden relief of abdominal pain followed by increased generalized pain in suspected appendicitis may

indicate an appendix rupture, which may lead to potentially fatal peritonitis.

2. A nasogastric tube may be used when appendicitis is complicated by peritonitis to decompress the stomach or alleviate GI symptoms.

3. After abdominal surgery, positive bowel sounds, passing of flatus (gas in the digestive tract), and bowel movements can be indicators of return of peristalsis (wavelike movement) and bowel function.

Precaution

If appendicitis is suspected, the patient should not be given laxatives or enemas, which will increase peristalsis and lead to appendix perforation. Nor should any heat compresses be applied to the abdomen; increased circulation can precipitate appendix rupture. Giving narcotics for pain relief before the diagnosis is made can mask signs of severity of the condition, such as appendix rupture.

BOTULISM

Botulism mostly results from consumption of inadequately cooked or improperly processed or preserved contaminated foods. The toxins caused by *Clostridium botulinum* (an anaerobic bacillus) will affect nerve function and lead to muscle paralysis. This infection is potentially fatal when the respiratory muscles are affected.

Main Symptoms

- Possible weakness, sore throat, vomiting, and diarrhea (without fever)
- Neurologic abnormalities including drooping of the eyelids or double vision (without affecting mental or sensory processes)
- Defective speech due to impairment of muscles essential to speech (dysarthria)

- Descending weakness of muscles in the trunk, arms, and legs
- Dyspnea caused by respiratory muscle paralysis

Selected Nursing Tips

1. If botulism is suspected, obtain a detailed dietary history of the patient and collect samples, if possible, to identify the toxin before administering antitoxin as prescribed.
2. If botulinum antitoxin is ordered, gather an accurate history of allergies (especially to horses) and perform a skin test as prescribed. Keep emergency supplies readily available for potential allergic reactions.
3. Assess and observe the patient for signs of neurologic symptoms, such as visual or speech disturbance.
4. Monitor fluid and electrolyte balance; report botulism cases as per protocol.

Points to Consider

1. Honey and corn syrup should not be fed to infants due to the possibility of their contamination with *C. botulinum* spores.
2. Isolation is not needed. Measures such as inducing vomiting or gastric lavage may be used to purge recently ingested unabsorbed toxins from the bowel as permitted or ordered.
3. Botulism resulting from wound infection is uncommon. Inadequately cooked and preserved foods are more likely to harbor the botulism pathogen.

Precaution

Avoid eating poorly preserved foods. Even "taste-testing" a bit of the content from a bulging can may prove lethal.

CHOLELITHIASIS AND CHOLECYSTITIS

In cholelithiasis, the stones or calculi are present in the gallbladder. The formation of gallstones often results from an imbalance of the bile components, though the precise etiology of this imbalance is often unclear. Infection or cholesterol-metabolism disturbance may alter the balance of bile composition. Gallstones are more likely to form when the bile cholesterol concentration is high and the flow is sluggish due to any of several reasons, such as immobility, diabetes mellitus, obesity, or rapid weight loss.

Gallstone incidence increases with age possibly due to the liver's increased synthesis of cholesterol and the decreased secretion of bile acid. However, elderly patients and some other individuals may not experience typical symptoms, such as fever, pain, or jaundice. Consequently, they may delay seeking necessary treatment, which increases their risk of complications.

Cholecystitis—that is, inflammation or infection of the gallbladder—is often associated with obstruction caused by gallstones or trauma.

Main Symptoms

Cholelithiasis may produce no symptoms or only mild GI discomfort. At other times, gallbladder attacks or biliary colic (pain and spasm resulting from bile duct obstruction by a gallstone), often precipitated by fatty meals, may present with any of the following symptoms:

- Excruciating pain (often recurrent) in the right upper quadrant of the abdomen, radiating to the back
- Fat intolerance, GI distress, and diaphoresis (profuse sweating)
- Jaundice (yellowish skin color) in some patients, when the common bile duct is obstructed and the bile is then absorbed in the blood (and bilirubin levels in the blood may be elevated)

Symptoms of acute cholecystitis may include upper right abdominal tenderness and rigidity with nausea/vomiting and signs of inflammation or infection, such as an increased white blood cell count and fever. When bile flow is obstructed, stools may become clay-colored, as the feces do not contain bile pigment.

When they have chronic cholecystitis, patients may experience symptoms such as recurrent heartburn or fat intolerance.

Selected Nursing Tips

1. Nursing management of acute cholecystitis is primarily directed toward relieving the patient's pain or spasm and removing or treating the cause. Monitor the patient for signs of complications, such as gallbladder perforation, peritonitis, and pancreatitis, and intervene as indicated.

2. Motivate the patient to participate in regular exercise or health-promoting activities, which may improve fat metabolism and aid in maintaining the desirable weight. Obesity is one of the risk factors of stone formation.

3. Avoiding excessive dietary intake of fat may decrease stimulation of the gallbladder and reduce the concentration of cholesterol in the bile, lowering the risk of gallstone formation.

Points to Consider

1. A low-fat diet and small, frequent meals are often better tolerated by patients with cholclithiasis. Fat stimulates gallbladder bile secretion; the bile flow in the duodenum of these patients may be impeded.

2. Ultrasound of the gallbladder is commonly used to assist with the diagnosis of gallbladder stones. Discouraging patients from drinking carbonated beverages prior to their tests to decrease intestinal gas may be necessary.

3. After food ingestion, the bile stored in the gallbladder is released into the small intestine (duodenum) to help with the digestion and fat absorption. When a patient's common

bile duct is obstructed, the decreased bile flow can affect the absorption of essential fatty acids and fat-soluble vitamins. Vitamin K deficiency increases the patient's tendency to bleed.

Precaution

In caring for a patient after cholecystectomy (gallbladder excision), report symptoms such as clay-colored stools, jaundice, dark yellow urine, fever, or abdominal pain. These symptoms may be indicators of serious complications.

CIRRHOSIS

The normal liver performs a multitude of essential functions: It secretes bile, stores fat-soluble vitamins and iron, detoxifies chemicals such as alcohol and medications, synthesizes proteins (e.g., clotting factors and albumin), and regulates glucose and bilirubin metabolism, among many other capabilities. In the progressive liver disease known as hepatic cirrhosis, normal liver tissue is often replaced with fibrotic tissue, causing degenerative changes and eventually affecting the liver's functions. This condition can be traced to diverse etiologies, including alcoholism and hepatitis.

Main Symptoms

Regardless of the specific cause, the symptoms of cirrhosis are often similar, resulting from the liver's failure to carry out its normal functions. This organ's functional deterioration may affect multiple systems, with manifestations including the following:

- Anemia and greater bleeding tendency due to the impaired ability of the liver to produce proteins (e.g., clotting factors, albumin).
- Gastric distress, such as anorexia, nausea, vomiting, constipation or diarrhea, and abdominal pain (possibly due to an enlarged liver).

- Mental changes (due to the involvement of the central nervous system), lethargy, slurred speech, confusion (due to an elevated serum ammonia level resulting from the liver's inability to convert ammonia into urea to be excreted), and signs of hepatic encephalopathy.
- Abdominal ascites (fluid accumulation in the peritoneal cavity) with inadequate gas exchange and hypoxia.
- Generalized weakness and fatigue due to possibly inadequate glucose supply. The liver stores carbohydrates as glycogen to be converted to glucose for use as needed; when this function is impaired, fatigue sets in.

Selected Nursing Tips

1. Nursing care approaches may include providing supportive care, managing symptoms, and minimizing complications.
2. Before administering a new medication to a patient with a liver disorder, consider its metabolic route.
3. In preparation for an invasive procedure, ensure the safety of the patient with liver disorder by assessing the results of coagulation studies, and address concerns as they arise.
4. Promoting rest may reduce metabolic demands on the liver; providing small, frequent meals and proper amounts of protein (consistent with the liver's function) as recommended may improve the patient's nutritional status.
5. In patients with fluid volume excess related to ascites, sodium and fluid intake may be limited as prescribed. Keeping records of daily weight, fluid intake/output, and abdominal girth can help monitor fluid status.
6. Avoidance of alcohol is essential to prevent further damage to the liver.
7. Identify and reduce the risks of bleeding. Advise patients to avoid activities that may increase abdominal pressure, such as straining or vigorous nose blowing; replace sharp objects, such as razors, with safer appliances (e.g., electric shavers). A patient with cirrhosis is susceptible to bleeding due to impaired liver production of clotting factors.

Points to Consider

1. Clay-colored stools can result from the liver's decreased ability to excrete bilirubin. Bilirubin—the yellowish bile pigment derived from hemoglobin of destroyed RBCs that have completed their life span—gives the feces its normal color. Jaundice may develop when serum bilirubin level is abnormally elevated, causing all the body tissues, including the sclerae and the skin, to appear greenish-yellow. The retained bilirubin (and bile salt) can irritate peripheral nerve endings, causing intense itching.

2. A low-protein diet is likely to be prescribed for a patient with cirrhosis or hepatic encephalopathy, in whom ammonia levels are elevated due to the liver's dysfunction related to protein metabolism and end-product excretion. Ammonia is formed from the decomposition of nitrogen-containing substances such as proteins and amino acids.

3. A patient with liver failure may have increased confusion due to the high serum level of ammonia. (When the liver fails to convert ammonia into urea to be excreted in the urine, the ammonia level rises.) Administration of prescribed lactulose (Cephulac) in patients with cirrhosis may lead to a decreased ammonia level, which lessens confusion.

Precaution

Liver damage can also be caused by an overdose of acetaminophen (Tylenol), or other hepatotoxic drugs, especially when combined with alcohol.

CLOSTRIDIUM DIFFICILE INFECTION

Clostridium difficile infection often manifests as diarrhea, and is frequently associated with the use of antibiotics. Any antibiotics, but especially broad-spectrum agents such as clindamycin (Cleocin), can destroy the beneficial microorganisms (normal flora) in the bowel along with the target bacteria, allowing *C. difficile* to flourish. Diarrhea can result from the toxins produced by *C. difficile*.

Main Symptoms

- Foul-smelling, unformed (or even grossly bloody) diarrhea
- Abdominal cramps
- Possibly fever and dehydration

Selected Nursing Tips

1. Instituting infection control precautions is essential in preventing and containing the spread of the pathogen. Meticulous hand washing is a must; the spores of the bacterium can be resistant to disinfectants and may be carried on the hands after contact with previously contaminated equipment.
2. Assessment should include asking the patient about the use of antibiotics or recent travel.
3. Judicious use of antibiotic therapy is important; identify the antibiotic possibly related to the condition and report it to the practitioner. Metronidazole (Flagyl), an antibiotic or antiprotozoal agent, may be prescribed if discontinuation of the causal antibiotic fails to relieve the patient's symptoms. Inform the patient that this medication may turn urine reddish-brown in color; alcohol-containing beverage should be avoided for at least a few days after the last dose.
4. Implement strict contact isolation. For example, the nurse might procure a disposable stethoscope for use with this patient only.

Point to Consider

Indiscriminate use of antibiotics is not beneficial. Hospitalized patients taking antibiotics are at a higher risk of developing infection with *C. difficile* (or multidrug-resistant strains of other bacteria).

Precaution

The *C. difficile* spores can survive on the surfaces of objects, such as commodes, telephones, and bedside tables, for a long period of time. The spores are heat resistant, and their presence is prevalent in healthcare facilities. Practicing thorough hand washing is an important infection-control step.

COLORECTAL CANCER

Manifestations of colorectal cancer—a malignant tumor in the colon or rectum—depend on the location, type, extent, and complications of the lesion. Incidence of this type of cancer is high in individuals with a family history. Consuming a diet high in animal products or processed foods and low in fiber increases the risk for developing colorectal cancer.

Main Symptoms

In many cases, clinical manifestations are not apparent in the early stages of colorectal cancer. When the disease becomes advanced, most patients experience symptoms such as the following:

- Melena (black, tarry stools) and rectal bleeding
- Abdominal pain or fullness, and change in bowel habits
- Anorexia, weakness, anemia, and weight loss

Lesions on the left-side descending colon tend to constrict the lumen, causing obstruction symptoms. These symptoms may include rectal bleeding, changes in bowel habits (e.g., abdominal pain or cramping, constipation, or ribbon-shaped stools), distension, or feeling of incomplete bowel movements.

Lesions on the right side are often asymptomatic because the stools in that part of the colon are more liquefied. Patients may have vague abdominal discomfort or melena. Fatigue and weakness may result from occult (hidden) bleeding or anemia.

Rectal lesions may produce symptoms including rectal pain, alternating constipation and diarrhea, and blood in the stool.

Selected Nursing Tips

1. Following a colon resection, assessing the patient for bowel sounds and passing of gas—both of which are signs of the return of peristalsis and normal GI function—is of high priority. The patient may experience pain caused by flatulence. Walking as tolerated may alleviate the "gas pain."

2. Polyps and inflammatory bowel disease can predispose patients to colorectal cancer. Because of its insidious onset, with symptoms appearing only in late-stage disease, regular colonoscopy per protocol is necessary to screen patients, remove polyps, and diagnose disease.

3. Rectal cancer may present with rectal bleeding, which can be an early sign. A simple way to screen for GI bleeding is a yearly fecal occult (hidden) blood test. Because other conditions (e.g., hemorrhoids) may also cause bleeding, further examination is needed if the test result is positive.

4. When more effective therapy cannot be rendered, alleviating pain and suffering are the focus of palliative care.

Points to Consider

1. To prevent colon cancer, a diet low in animal fat and high in fiber, including vegetables, fruits, and grains, is recommended. The metabolic end-products of a high-fat diet may be carcinogenic. A lack of bulk in the diet decreases GI motility and prolongs the passage of the stools in the intestinal tract, thereby lengthening exposure to possible carcinogens. Chronic use of tobacco or alcohol also increases the risk of colorectal cancer.

2. If colostomy is indicated, prepare the patient and the family for lifestyle adjustment and proper stoma care.

Precaution

Whenever rectal bleeding occurs, it is important to rule out possible cancer, even if the patient has known hemorrhoids or diverticular disease.

CONSTIPATION/FECAL IMPACTION

Multiple factors are implicated in the development of constipation, which is defined as a decrease and difficulty in having bowel movements. This condition can result from insufficient dietary fiber or fluid intake, physical inactivity, many medications (such as antibiotics and opioids), and various disease processes that slow GI transit or affect neurologic function.

Unresolved constipation, especially in bedridden and elderly patients or after barium administration (orally or rectally), may lead to fecal impaction. Such impaction has serious consequences.

Main Symptoms

Patients with constipation may have abdominal discomfort or distension, and may strain to pass stools. When hard stools have impacted the bowel, the patient may, instead, experience oozing mucus or watery feces, mimicking diarrhea. This sign should be taken seriously and addressed. Nausea and projectile vomiting may also occur.

Selected Nursing Tips

1. Encourage patients to increase their fluid and dietary fiber intake. The fiber and bulk in fruits and vegetables can stimulate peristalsis and facilitate bowel movements.
2. Motivate or assist patients—especially elderly and disabled people—to incorporate moderate and appropriate exercise into their daily routines.
3. Advise patients to maintain a routine bowel schedule and promptly respond to the urge to defecate. Educate them to avoid overuse of habit-forming laxatives.
4. For fecal impaction, an enema may be prescribed to soften hardened feces. Manual removal by a lubricated gloved finger may also be necessary, per protocol or order.

Points to Consider

1. Habitual suppression of the urge to move the bowels may cause the rectal muscles to be less sensitive to the presence

of the feces. In addition, owing to water absorption, the longer the stools are retained in the rectum, the harder and drier it becomes, making defecation more difficult.

2. Bulk-forming laxatives, such as psyllium, must be taken with adequate (at least 240 mL) liquid to prevent serious adverse effects, because such products will swell.

3. Prolonged use of laxatives tends to inhibit a normal bowel pattern and can cause the colon to become dilated and atonic (lacking muscle tone), creating a feeling of constipation and contributing to the perpetual use of laxatives.

Precautions

1. If patients have vascular problems, such as heart failure or high blood pressure, constipation and straining may potentially cause a medical emergency such as a coronary event. Advise the patient to take measures to prevent constipation.

2. During or after digital removal of stools, monitor the patient's heart rate, as vagal stimulation can cause bradycardia (a slow heart rate).

3. Prolonged bowel obstruction can cause serious complications, including perforation and gangrene.

DIVERTICULOSIS AND DIVERTICULITIS

A diverticulum is a bulging pouch of the intestinal mucosae. In diverticulosis, multiple non-inflamed diverticula are present in the GI tract.

Diverticulitis differs from diverticulosis in that there is inflammation of the diverticula in the former condition.

Main Symptoms

Diverticulosis may be asymptomatic. In some cases, it may cause abdominal pain, which is accompanied by alternating constipation and diarrhea. The pain is often relieved by passing of flatus or having bowel movements.

Patients with diverticulitis may present with symptoms of infection, including leukocytosis (increased serum white blood cell count) and low-grade fever, in addition to nausea, vomiting, or dull abdominal pain with irregular bowel habits.

Selected Nursing Tips

1. Recommend a diet high in fiber, such as fruits and vegetables, and low in fat and red meat. Advocate regular exercise and weight reduction (in obese persons), which may reduce the risk of developing diverticulosis.

2. Advise patients to avoid straining at stools, bending, lifting, or wearing tight, restrictive clothing to prevent increasing intraabdominal pressure, which may precipitate an attack.

3. Bowel rest, a liquid diet, or parenteral fluids may be ordered during an acute episode. Barium enema or other procedures that can pose risks for perforation and peritonitis in patients with acute diverticulitis are usually avoided.

4. In those rare cases in which the condition cannot be managed medically, provide education and postoperative/ostomy care as indicated.

Points to Consider

1. The development of diverticula is often attributed to consumption of a low-fiber diet, because the lack of bulk predisposes individuals to constipation. A longer transit time in the intestines causes more water to be absorbed from the stools, contributing to formation of diverticula. Retention of undigested food with bacteria in the diverticula may be implicated in the development of diverticulitis.

2. Diverticula can potentially cause obstruction, perforation, infection, or bleeding. In severe cases of diverticulitis, abscesses or peritonitis may develop with symptoms including abdominal rigidity, pain, diminished intestinal motility, and retention of air, fluid, and stools.

3. Chronic diverticulitis occasionally may cause the inflamed colon segment to adhere to the bladder or other organs, producing a fistula.

Precaution

Small, poorly digestible foods are best avoided by patients with these conditions. For example, foods such as popcorn, nuts, or some seeds can get stuck in diverticular pouches (though a causal relationship has not been statistically established).

GASTRIC (STOMACH) CANCER

Although the exact causative agent of stomach cancer has not been identified and the etiology remains unknown, predisposing factors for this disease are believed to include chronic gastric inflammation, ulcer, atrophy, infection with *Helicobacter pylori* bacteria, and other conditions that cause mucosal injury. Certain kinds of food preparation or preservation (e.g., smoking, salting, or pickling), as well as tobacco use or high alcohol intake, may also be implicated in the development of gastric cancer.

Main Symptoms

Early presenting symptoms of stomach cancer are often vague or nonspecific. Patients' complaints or symptoms may vary, but include the following manifestations:

- Early satiety after meal with abdominal discomfort or fullness
- Poor appetite and weight loss
- Anemia, fatigue, and lethargy

Some patients may have dysphagia (difficulty in swallowing) or coffee-ground vomitus. Occult (hidden) blood tests of stools may be positive. However, there are no symptoms that are considered specifically diagnostic for stomach cancer.

Selected Nursing Tips

1. Provide adequate nutrition and necessary (i.e., prescribed) vitamin supplementation to correct nutritional deficits secondary to gastric cancer before and after the surgery.

The stomach contains cells that secrete intrinsic factor for vitamin B_{12} absorption. After a total gastrectomy, routine B_{12} supplementation is needed to prevent pernicious anemia.

2. After gastrectomy surgery, assist the patient in frequent coughing, turning, and deep breathing at proper intervals to prevent respiratory compromise, which often occurs postoperatively.

3. Explain to the postoperative patient that use of an incentive spirometer as ordered helps the lungs to expand, thereby reducing the risk of pulmonary complications.

4. Assist the patient to assume a proper position as prescribed (such as semi-Fowler's position or semi-sitting position) that facilitates breathing and drainage, but does not cause too much fatigue.

5. Take measures to minimize the side effects (e.g., nausea or vomiting) of the treatment, which may include chemotherapy or radiation therapy.

Points to Consider

After undergoing gastric resection, some patients may develop dumping syndrome. This syndrome commonly occurs after meals when there is no stomach to hold all the intake, so that ingested food rapidly enters the small intestine before being properly processed. In turn, the higher osmotic pressure pulls fluid into the bowel lumen, decreasing blood volume. The patient may experience physiological alterations, including dizziness, palpitation, weakness, sweating, abdominal cramping, or the urge to defecate. The symptoms will subside or resolve over time.

To manage dumping syndrome, recommend the following measures to help minimize the effects:

- Consume small, frequent meals with moderate amounts of protein and fat; avoid foods high in simple sugars.

- Drink liquids between meals, but not with meals. If fluid is added to ingested food, rapid emptying of the stomach contents into the small intestine is likely to occur, thereby aggravating the dumping syndrome.
- Lying down after eating, if not contraindicated, may slow the passage of the ingested food into the small intestine.

Precaution

After stomach surgery, avoid irrigating or manipulating the nasogastric (NG) tube, because doing so may increase the pressure at the incision site and potentially cause rupture.

GASTROENTERITIS

Gastroenteritis is a general term used to describe irritation and inflammation of the GI lining. Other terms are more appropriate when specific causes are identified. The causative agents can be bacteria, viruses, parasites, toxins, or others.

Although gastroenteritis is often self-limiting, it can be debilitating or life-threatening, especially in elderly or infirm patients.

Main Symptoms

- Diarrhea and abdominal discomfort—universal characteristics of the syndrome
- Anorexia
- Nausea and vomiting

Selected Nursing Tips

1. Nursing assessment should include obtaining a diet history so as to identify the cause and determine the appropriate treatment.
2. Once the diagnosis is established, contact precautions should be implemented; thorough hand washing should be practiced as a universal precaution.

3. Withhold food or fluid until vomiting subsides to prevent aspiration.
4. Dehydration can be a great concern due to excessive loss of fluids and electrolytes through diarrhea or vomiting. Dry mucous membranes, poor skin turgor, sunken eyes, lethargy, oliguria, substantial weight loss, and fever may be signs of dehydration, which is a serious complication. Muscle weakness or cramping may be a sign of hypokalemia resulting from excessive diarrhea. Careful rehydration and electrolyte maintenance are essential. Report food poisoning cases to the local public health authorities and take a sample of the contaminated food, if possible, in anticipation of further investigation.

Points to Consider

1. Infection caused by bacteria such as *Salmonella* may occur after eating undercooked or contaminated foods. Manifestations may include diarrhea, nausea, vomiting, abdominal cramping, and possibly low-grade fever or weakness.
2. Whereas excessive vomiting is likely to cause metabolic alkalosis due to the loss of hydrochloric acid, severe diarrhea may lead to metabolic acidosis because of the excretion of bicarbonate.

Precaution

To prevent food poisoning, refrigerating all meats and dairy products properly is an important step, as bacteria thrive in a warm, moist environment.

GASTROESOPHAGEAL REFLUX DISEASE

In gastroesophageal reflux disease (GERD), there is a backflow of acidic gastric contents into the esophagus without associated vomiting or belching. GERD may result from a variety of conditions. It can also occur when the lower esophageal sphincter (LES) is unable to create sufficient pressure to close the lower end of the esophagus normally, or when the pressure within the stomach is higher than the LES pressure. The refluxed acidic gastric contents can cause irritation or inflammation of the esophagus.

Predisposing factors for GERD include conditions or positions that increase intra-abdominal pressure, such as hiatal hernia, bending, and the use/intake of substances that reduce LES control, such as cigarettes, alcohol, certain drugs, or fatty foods.

Main Symptoms

- Indigestion (dyspepsia), heartburn, and noncardiac chest pain that worsens after meals and is relieved with antacids or by sitting up
- Pain on swallowing (dysphagia)
- Regurgitation and bloating after eating

Selected Nursing Tips

1. Encourage patients to eat small, frequent meals and drink fluids between meals to prevent stomach distension; avoid substances or foods that reduce LES tone, including tobacco, alcohol, caffeine, certain medications, and fatty, spicy, or acidic foods.
2. Sitting up after meals and sleeping with the head of the bed elevated can help minimize reflux.
3. Help patients with GERD to maintain their ideal weight. Being overweight increases abdominal pressure, which increases the tendency to reflux.
4. Advise patients to avoid activities that compress the abdomen and increase intra-abdominal pressure, including bending, lifting, or wearing tight clothing.

Points to Consider

1. The symptoms of GERD may be minimized by avoiding circumstances that increase intra-abdominal pressure, neutralizing gastric acid contents, and strengthening the LES with preventive means, drugs or, in extremely severe cases, with surgical interventions.

2. Excessive dietary fat may decrease esophageal sphincter tone or increase weight, thereby increasing the risk for GERD.

3. Symptoms of GERD vary from person to person. Some may be atypical, such as chronic cough, sore throat, hoarseness, and asthma.

4. Bariatric surgery has been used in treating morbid obesity and maintaining sustained weight loss in many individuals, but not without certain undesirable effects. In some surgeries, the weight loss goal is primarily achieved through either reducing stomach size to curb food intake or bypassing portions of the small intestine to decrease the absorption of ingested food. Using a combination of the two approaches is common. Less invasive bariatric procedures based on different mechanisms are also available.

Precaution

Persistent reflux may cause complications such as esophagitis due to the direct effects of gastric acid on the esophageal mucosa.

HEPATITIS, VIRAL

Hepatitis refers to inflammation of the liver, which is frequently caused by a virus (as in hepatitis A, B, C, D, E, or G). Other nonviral causative agents or conditions include toxins, alcohol, drug (e.g., acetaminophen) overdose, and autoimmune liver disease.

Acute hepatitis A is highly contagious. The pathogen is usually transmitted via the fecal-oral route, through ingesting food or water contaminated with hepatitis A virus, or through close contact with carriers of the virus. The hepatitis E virus is also transmitted by the fecal-oral and waterborne routes, commonly through drinking contaminated water.

The hepatitis B, C, and D viruses are commonly transmitted via exposure to infected blood or body secretions. The hepatitis G virus can be transmitted through a bloodborne route such as blood transfusion.

Main Symptoms

The incubation periods of the different types of viral hepatitis may vary. The presentation of hepatitis A may resemble that of a flu infection. Most patients with viral hepatitis experience the following symptoms, which may or may not include jaundice (icterus):

- Easy fatigue and weakness
- GI symptoms such as anorexia, nausea, and occasional vomiting
- Malaise, flulike symptoms, and low-grade fever
- Dark-colored urine due to bilirubin being excreted in the urine, and clay-colored stools if the bile ducts are obstructed or inflamed
- Skin rash and pruritus (itching)
- Pain in the right upper quadrant of the abdomen or in the joints

Clinical assessment findings may include hepatomegaly (enlarged liver) upon physical examination and elevated serum liver-enzyme levels.

Selected Nursing Tips

1. Currently, there is no specific therapy for most viral hepatitis. Emphasis is placed on provision of adequate nutrition and rest to facilitate the liver's regeneration.
2. Ensure patients' rest periods by carefully scheduling nursing procedures and patient activities. During the acute phase of hepatitis, the patient is usually placed on bed rest to reduce metabolic demands and lessen fatigue, which is a common complaint in patients with cellular damage of the liver.
3. Provide adequate nutrition through small, frequent meals; correct fluid and electrolyte imbalances. Encourage the patient, if appropriate, to consume the largest meal in the morning, when it may be better tolerated. In general, patients with hepatitis need to increase their fluid intake, including fruit juices for anorectic patients.

4. Enteral isolation precautions should be instituted to prevent transmission of hepatitis A and E. Hand washing, especially after using the bathroom, should be stressed. Hepatitis cases, like many other infectious diseases, should be reported to public health authorities per protocol.
5. Standard precautions should be practiced with all patients. Advise patients not to share personal items such as razors, pierced earrings, and toothbrushes.

Points to Consider

1. Many drugs are potentially hepatotoxic. Improper use of over-the-counter medications containing acetaminophen has been linked to acute liver failure.
2. Vaccination is an effective way to prevent hepatitis A or B infection. An antibody test is available to assist with the diagnosis of hepatitis C in some patients, but has less than ideal accuracy.
3. Patients with liver disease may have jaundice, resulting from accumulation of bilirubin in the blood; jaundice may result from various pathologies, including bilirubin release due to liver cell injury by viruses or toxins.
4. Before discharge, counsel the patient to avoid alcohol or alcohol-containing substances and to take measures to prevent recurrence of hepatitis.
5. Nursing interventions for a patient with toxic hepatitis often focus on alleviating the patient's symptoms and discomfort in addition to removing the causative agent.

Precautions

1. Instruct patients to report clay-colored stools, which may indicate hepatic bile obstruction.
2. Using defective gloves may result in the healthcare provider contracting hepatitis B through contact with the patient's body fluids.

HIATAL HERNIA

A hernia is an abnormal protrusion of an organ through a weakening of the wall; a hiatus is an opening. In hiatal hernia, the diaphragm opening, through which the esophagus passes, becomes abnormally enlarged, allowing the stomach to move up into the chest cavity.

The exact cause of hiatal hernia has yet to be determined. This condition often arises when the diaphragm muscle weakens due to aging or other conditions associated with trauma or increased intra-abdominal pressure, including obesity, tumors, tight girdle or garments, and intense physical exertion.

The symptoms of hiatal hernia may occur when the patient lies down after a meal, causing intra-abdominal pressure to increase. The stomach usually returns to the abdominal cavity when the patient returns to an upright position.

Hernia can give rise to serious complications, including hemorrhage, obstruction, or strangulation in some cases.

Main Symptoms

- Heartburn or chest pain worsened by reclining, resembling that in other conditions, such as angina or GERD
- Regurgitation
- Belching and dysphagia

Patients with an intact LES may exhibit no symptoms.

Selected Nursing Tips

1. Conservative therapy involves lifestyle modifications to eliminate causes or triggers. Patients with hiatal hernia are recommended to eat small, frequent meals that can easily pass through the esophagus. In addition, they should avoid alcohol, smoking, and activities involving physical straining.
2. Sitting up or elevating the head of the bed after eating may help keep the stomach in the abdominal cavity.

3. Symptoms of hiatal hernia can usually be managed with medication as well as diet and lifestyle changes, such as weight reduction.
4. Emergency surgery will be indicated when the hernia causes the blood flow to the area or intestine to be restricted.

Point to Consider

Hiatal hernia may recur after surgical repair. Anti-reflux surgeries are commonly performed laparoscopically with specific nursing care guidelines.

Precautions

1. After gastric surgery, monitor NG tube patency to prevent stomach distension, which can cause a breakdown of the repair. The NG tube should not be manipulated. If it is malfunctioning, report that problem to the practitioner.
2. A reducible hernia can be reduced back into place, whereas an "incarcerated" hernia is an irreducible hernia. Emergency intervention is indicated to treat incarcerated hernia and prevent strangulation, which may restrict the blood flow to the area and result in serious complications if not immediately corrected, including pain, tissue necrosis of the herniated portion of the stomach, and shock.

INFLAMMATORY BOWEL DISEASE: CROHN'S DISEASE AND ULCERATIVE COLITIS

Chronic inflammatory bowel disease (IBD) includes both Crohn's disease and ulcerative colitis. These conditions involve chronic bowel inflammation at various sites to varying degrees. The exact cause of IBD is unclear.

IBD is characterized by severe diarrhea and abdominal pain with periods of remission and exacerbation. Possible triggers and exacerbating factors may include stress, other illnesses, and exposure to harmful chemicals or substances, including tobacco or radiation.

Main Symptoms

The terminal ileum is frequently the site of Crohn's disease, though any portion of the GI tract can be affected, including all layers. Inflammatory lesions are segmental and subject to remission and exacerbation. The bowel inflammation associated with Crohn's disease may cause increased peristalsis and cramping with the following manifestations:

- Usually nonbloody severe diarrhea, steatorrhea (fatty stools), and flatulence
- Abdominal cramping pain, often in the right lower quadrant, which worsens after meals
- Intermittent low-grade fever and malaise
- Malabsorption and malnutrition with weight loss
- Possible perianal fistulas or abscesses or urinary tract infection resulting from a bowel/bladder fistula (an abnormal tube-like passage), with feces sometimes seen in urine

In ulcerative colitis, inflammation usually originates from the rectum and the descending colon on the left side, with the potential for spreading continuously throughout the entire length of the colon. This condition often affects the innermost mucosal layer of the bowel wall, so fistulas are rare. Depending on the severity of the disease, manifestations may include the following signs and symptoms:

- Frequent bloody stools (up to 10–20 times per day) or rectal bleeding, and possibly anemia
- Abdominal bloating or pain, which is intensified with stress or after meals, and is often relieved with passage of stools or gas
- Fever during acute attacks

Comparison of Crohn's Disease and Ulcerative Colitis

	Crohn's Disease	**Ulcerative Colitis**
Pattern of inflammation	Segmental, anywhere in GI tract, mostly in the terminal ileum, involving all layers; may cause fistulas, abscesses, or strictures	Continuously from the rectum up, often involving the inner mucosa layer of the colon; fistulas are rare
Diarrhea	Mostly nonbloody	Often bloody with mucus
Abdominal cramping pain	Common, colicky	Common
Intermittent fever	Common	During acute phase
Weight loss	Can be severe	Less common
Nutritional deficiencies	Common	Less common
Toxic megacolon	Uncommon	More common

Selected Nursing Tips

1. Evaluate patients with IBD for signs of fluid and electrolyte imbalances, such as muscle cramping (a sign of a low blood potassium level), which could lead to a dangerous cardiac dysrhythmia.
2. Hydration and nutritional support are necessary to address possible weight loss; set a realistic and measurable weight-gain goal and encourage the patient to follow through on achieving it.
3. Vitamin supplementation may be prescribed to patients with IBD due to inadequate vitamin absorption in their intestines.
4. During exacerbations, a low-residual (low-fiber) diet may be preferred because it reduces bowel movement frequency and

is less irritating to the bowel. Consult the dietician regarding individualized dietary recommendations to meet the patient's nutritional needs. Note that beverages containing caffeine can be chemically irritating to the intestinal mucosa.

5. Surgery is often reserved for certain severe complications, including bowel perforation, obstruction, and hemorrhage. The nursing priority after ostomy surgery includes having the patient demonstrate competency in safely managing ostomy care.

6. Emotional stress can adversely impact the disease process, whereas stress reduction is conducive to alleviation of the symptoms of IBD.

Points to Consider

1. Sulfasalazine (Azulfidine) may decrease the inflammatory response. When this drug is administered, ensure adequate fluid intake and monitor for side effects (e.g., nausea, vomiting, and anorexia). Watch for signs of hypersensitivity to the medication.

2. Patients with ulcerative colitis disease are at risk for developing toxic megacolon, an extremely dilated segment of the colon resulting from partial bowel paralysis.

3. Parenteral nutrition (PN) therapy may be used to meet patients' nutritional needs when indicated. The total parenteral nutrition (TPN) solution is specifically mixed based on the individual's condition. It is administered intravenously through a large central vein, such as a subclavian vein. The increased blood flow in a large vein can adequately dilute a highly concentrated solution. Strict adherence to the TPN administration guidelines is critical. Ensure the correct rate of administration, and monitor for signs of hyperglycemia (high blood sugar), as the TPN solution is often high in glucose. Subsequently, overproduction of insulin or administration of excessive doses of insulin to counteract the high glucose level can lead to hypoglycemia (low blood sugar),

which also requires immediate nursing intervention. Monitor lab results, weight, intake/output, and blood sugar closely as per the nursing protocol.

Precaution

Manage fluid, electrolytes, and nutritional imbalances. Monitor for signs of complications, such as bleeding (likely in ulcerative colitis) or small bowel obstruction (possibly in Crohn's disease).

ORAL CANCER

Oral cancer is uncontrollable cell growth on the lips or anywhere in the mouth. The definitive cause of this malignancy is not clear. Predisposing factors may include tobacco use in any form; excessive alcohol intake; chronic irritation, including eating hot or spicy foods; and mechanical problems, such as poor dental alignment. Squamous cell carcinoma is a common type. Treatment may include surgery, radiation, chemotherapy, or a combination of these modalities. Early detection and treatment are key to successful patient outcomes.

Main Symptoms

- Initially, a nonhealing lesion on the lips or mouth, which may be hardened, painless, whitish or reddish, inflamed, and irregularly shaped
- Feeling of a lump in the neck, or complaining of sore throat or voice change
- Pain and difficulty in swallowing, chewing, or speaking, in later stages
- Enlarged cervical nodes and blood-tinged sputum

Laryngeal cancer may cause symptoms including hoarseness, a feeling of a foreign body in the throat, or difficulty swallowing.

Selected Nursing Tips

1. Any oral ulceration that does not respond to treatment should be evaluated further. A thickened white patch on

the tongue or nonhealing ulcers in the mouth should raise suspicion for oral cancer.

2. Assess the patient's support system. Provide teaching to the patient and the family prior to the treatment and explain the care required. If indicated, offer alternative means of communication (e.g., a writing pad) for temporary or permanent use.

3. Postoperatively, ensure airway patency and clearance. Perform care as prescribed, including suctioning gently as needed. Advise the patient to avoid hot or highly seasoned foods and commercial mouthwashes containing alcohol.

4. Chewing sugarless candy or sucking on ice chips may help alleviate mouth dryness—a frequent side effect of radiation therapy.

5. Enteral feedings or other means may be prescribed to meet patients' nutritional needs. Monitor the patient's intake and output; obtain daily weights using the same scale at the same time.

Points to Consider

1. Smoking or chewing tobacco, drinking alcohol, or even chronic irritation of a mechanical nature, such as an ill-fitting tooth, could make patients susceptible to developing oral cancer.

2. Use of both alcohol and tobacco further increases the risk of developing oral cancer due to these substances' synergistic carcinogenic effect. Patient education regarding reducing high-risk behaviors is one of nurses' important functions.

Precaution

Postoperatively, take precautions to prevent aspiration; airway obstruction can be a complication that requires immediate intervention.

PANCREATITIS

Pancreatitis involves inflammation of the pancreas, which may occur in acute or chronic form. Some cases of acute pancreatitis are mild and self-limiting, whereas others may evolve into a severe form of pancreatitis with significant or long-duration, life-threatening complications.

The pancreas serves as both an endocrine gland and an exocrine gland. In its role as an endocrine gland, the alpha cells and beta cells of its islets of Langerhans secrete glucagon and insulin, respectively. In its role as an exocrine gland, the pancreas secretes enzymes such as lipase, amylase, and trypsinogen (an inactive form of trypsin or a proenzyme that is converted to trypsin in the intestine), which are needed for digestion of fat, starch, and some proteins.

Pancreatitis often occurs after the pancreas has sustained injury. As a result, the pancreatic enzymes are activated prematurely within the pancreas (instead of in the intestines), causing self-digestion of the pancreas, although the underlying pathogenic mechanism is not well understood.

Numerous etiologic factors have been implicated in the development of this disease:

- Chronic alcohol ingestion
- Biliary (pertaining to bile) tract disorders
- Injury to the pancreatic cells
- Certain drugs, such as glucocorticoids or excessive use of acetaminophen
- Environmental and genetic factors
- Idiopathic (unknown) causes

Main Symptoms

Patients with acute pancreatitis often appear very sick and restless, exhibiting symptoms such as the following:

- A sudden-onset, steady, intense abdominal (and back) pain, which is not relieved by vomiting, and is aggravated by eating, lying flat, or walking

- Low-grade fever, vomiting, malaise, restlessness, and diaphoresis
- Hypotension, hypoxia, and dyspnea, reflecting potential complications such as sepsis or shock
- Alterations in laboratory and other test findings, such as an elevated white blood cell (WBC) count and increased serum amylase or lipase levels

Patients with chronic pancreatitis may exhibit the following clinical manifestations:

- Increasingly frequent abdominal and back pain, which is not relieved with food or antacids
- Weight loss and steatorrhea (frothy, foul-smelling stools due to malabsorption of fats)
- Hyperglycemia (reflecting pancreatic endocrine insufficiency)

Selected Nursing Tips

1. Acute pancreatitis is life-threatening emergency requiring vigorous supportive care. Monitor vital signs and intake/output; maintain electrolyte and fluid balance to prevent complications including potentially fatal shock. Be vigilant for signs and symptoms such as fever, cardiac irregularities, changes in lab values, and altered respiration patterns.
2. Nothing by mouth (NPO) status and placement of a naso-gastric tube may be ordered to decrease stimulation of the pancreas and relieve abdominal distension.
3. Pain relief is also a primary concern. Patients may find that assuming a comfortable position, such as sitting up or leaning forward, slightly mitigates the pain.
4. Observe the patient's respiratory status; proper and frequent changes in position as well as coughing or deep breathing may help prevent respiratory complications.
5. Monitor patients for electrolyte imbalances; watch for signs of a low blood calcium level (e.g., muscle twitching, jerking, numbness, tingling, or irritability).

6. During discharge teaching, the patient should be instructed to avoid alcohol and caffeine. Chronic use of alcohol could be the causative agent for pancreatitis, and caffeine is a stimulant that can irritate the pancreas.

Points to Consider

1. Identifying and treating the underlying causes of pancreatitis may help predict and manage complications and prevent recurrent attacks.
2. Patients with chronic pancreatitis may take prescribed pancreatic enzymes with a liberal amount of liquid when they have meals or snacks to facilitate digestion and prevent steatorrhea.

Precautions

1. Advocate avoidance of binge drinking, which can precipitate an acute episode of pancreatitis.
2. In some cases, to meet the patient's nutritional needs without causing discomfort associated with ingesting foods, parenteral nutrition therapy may be prescribed if the enteral route is not feasible. In such a case, it is critical to ensure an accurate infusion rate and monitor for signs of complications. Rapid infusion can cause intravascular fluid or glucose overload. Check the patient's glucose level to rule out hyperglycemia if indicated; administer insulin as prescribed.

PEPTIC ULCER DISEASE

In peptic ulcer disease (PUD), there is an erosion or ulcer of the GI mucosa. The specific condition may be termed gastric, duodenal, esophageal, or stress-related ulcer, depending on its location and causes. Peptic ulcers are now thought to be caused by infection with the bacterium *Helicobacter pylori* in many people who are predisposed to ulcer formation. There are different opinions and theories as to the causes of stress ulcers. Excessive secretion of gastric hydrochloric acid (HCl) or pepsin (digestive juice enzyme) may decrease mucosal resistance to bacteria; stress may be implicated in this condition. Inadequate blood flow to the gastric mucosa can cause mucosal break-down, thereby contributing to PUD.

Risk factors for PUD include consumption of offensive substances (e.g., alcohol, tobacco smoke, caffeinated beverages, or spicy foods), physiologic stress (e.g., burns, trauma), and use of certain medications (e.g., steroids or chronic use of nonsteroidal anti-inflammatory drugs [NSAIDs]).

Some ulcers may be reversed when patients recover from the stressful events. In general, however, PUD tends to be chronic, being marked by remissions and exacerbations.

Main Symptoms

- Gnawing or dull pain felt in the upper abdomen or back
- Pain high in the upper gastric area, often constant and intensified by eating, and early satiety (in gastric ulcer)
- Dull, "hunger-like" pain in the mid-epigastric area or in the back (in duodenal ulcer), especially when the stomach is empty, which may be alleviated by taking food or antacids to neutralize and dilute the HCl

Selected Nursing Tips

1. Counsel patients to reduce stress and avoid irritating foods or substances, including alcohol, smoking, caffeine, and, if possible, certain medications, such as NSAIDs, to minimize exacerbations.
2. Dietary management of patients with PUD may include having frequent, small meals or snacks at regular intervals to mix food with gastric acid and minimize mucosal irritation.
3. Administer medications according to the recommended schedule. Antacids can neutralize gastric acid and lessen the pain caused by peptic ulcer. To reduce the chances of drug interactions, antacids should not be taken with other medications.

4. When a patient with *H. pylori* infection is prescribed a combination of three medications—for example, metronidazole (Flagyl), an antibacterial/antiprotozoal agent; lansoprazole (Prevacid), a proton pump inhibitor; and another antibiotic medication, such as tetracycline—the nurse should emphasize the importance of completing the full drug regimen in an effort to eradicate the bacteria.

Points to Consider

1. It is recommended that proton-pump inhibitors that suppress gastric acid secretion, such as esomeprazole (Nexium) and lansoprazole (Prevacid), be taken prior to eating for better absorption. Ranitidine (Zantac), a histamine H_2 receptor antagonist and an antiulcer medication, is better given with meals or at bedtime. Antacids taken after ingestion of food may prolong their neutralizing effect.

2. Identifying and removing the causal factors for PUD can prove beneficial. Substances such as NSAIDs (e.g., aspirin) that inhibit prostaglandin synthesis may cause increased gastric acid secretion and decreased secretion of mucosa-protecting mucus; thus, their use may contribute to the development of PUD.

Precaution

Upper GI tract bleeding—a potential complication of peptic ulcer—may manifest as dark coffee-colored vomitus or black, tarry stools (resulting from digested hemoglobin). Nursing interventions may include monitoring oxygen saturation, administering oxygen, and establishing peripheral IV access for parenteral administration as per protocol or orders.

PERITONITIS

In peritonitis, the inflammation or infection of the peritoneum (the serous membrane that covers the abdominal organs and lines the abdominal cavity) can be either local or general, and either acute or chronic. Peritonitis can result from an array of pathologies. Secondary peritonitis is often caused by perforation of the abdominal organs, such as ruptured appendix; the resulting bacterial contamination of the usually sterile peritoneal cavity leads to fluid shifting to the peritoneal space and hypovolemia (decreased blood volume). This condition can be fatal if not treated promptly and effectively.

Main Symptoms

Clinical manifestations depend on the severity or extent of the infection, but may include the following symptoms:

- A sudden, severe abdominal pain and distension with rebound tenderness
- "Board-like" abdominal rigidity due to the intestinal obstruction, and decreased or absent bowel sounds due to loss of intestinal motility or paralytic ileus
- High fever and diaphoresis
- Nausea, vomiting, weakness, and pallor
- Dehydration, tachycardia, and hypotension

Selected Nursing Tips

1. NPO (nothing by mouth) status is usually instituted until the precipitating cause of peritonitis is treated. Surgical intervention is commonly required when perforation is the cause; this procedure seeks to remove the infectious material, drain accumulated fluid, and minimize the contamination.
2. Replace fluids and electrolytes and treat infection with antibiotics as ordered. The patient may need intensive care, IV analgesics, and nasogastric decompression as supportive measures. The nursing focus includes maintaining hemodynamic stability and combating infection to prevent peritonitis from advancing to shock and organ failure.
3. After surgery, provide standard and specific care as required; monitor the patient for the return of peristalsis by assessing for bowel sounds and passing of gas or bowel

movements. Teach the patient how to splint the incision to effectively breathe or cough; use an incentive spirometer frequently to aid in lung expansion and to prevent pulmonary complications.

Point to Consider

Early ambulation, as appropriate, may facilitate the return of bowel function and prevent postoperative complications and clot formation from immobility.

Precaution

Postoperatively, closely monitor the patient for signs of complications, including evisceration (spilling out of abdominal contents as a result of wound dehiscence or bursting open) and abscess formation.

CHAPTER 8

Genitourinary Issues

The genitourinary system encompasses either a female or a male reproductive system and the urinary system, which consists of two kidneys, two ureters, a urinary bladder, and a urethra.

The kidneys are the main organs of the urinary system. They perform several functions essential for the preservation of life. The kidneys filter the blood to maintain internal homeostasis; they also excrete into the urine what is not reabsorbed by the tubules as well as metabolic wastes such as urea (an end product of protein metabolism formed from ammonia), creatinine (an end product formed when phosphocreatine is used for muscle contraction) and uric acid (an end product of purine metabolism). Urine is produced by the kidneys through an extremely complex process, involving glomerular filtration, tubular reabsorption, and tubular secretion. The filtration process requires adequate blood volume and cardiac output.

The kidneys filter the blood through glomeruli, which are semipermeable membranes. Normally, the pores in the glomerular membranes are small enough to keep blood cells, platelets, and large plasma proteins from being filtered out. When capillary permeability is increased, as occurs in many diseases, plasma proteins and blood cells may pass into and be found in the urine. Glomerular filtration rate (GFR) refers to the amount of blood filtered by the glomeruli in a minute (or in a given time). GFR may serve as an indicator of the kidney's filtering capacity. (GFR is commonly measured by a creatinine clearance test, optimally based on a 24-hour urine collection.)

The kidneys also function to help regulate the body's acid–base balance through processes such as bicarbonate reabsorption and acid secretion. With the right amount of aldosterone and antidiuretic hormone (ADH), healthy kidneys can maintain fluid and electrolyte balance through excretion of the right amounts of ingested electrolytes, and regulate blood pressure. ADH, also known as vasopressin, and aldosterone play important roles in the renal reabsorption of water and sodium.

In concert with the liver, the kidneys can turn inactive forms of vitamin D into an active form to facilitate the absorption of calcium from the gastrointestinal (GI) tract. Inactive vitamin D is usually obtained in the diet or produced via the action of sunlight on cholesterol found in the skin.

The kidneys also produce erythropoietin, a hormone that stimulates the production of red blood cells (RBCs) in the bone marrow. In renal failure, a deficiency of erythropoietin may lead to anemia.

Renin, an enzyme produced from the renal cells, can convert angiotensinogen (a serum globulin fraction) to angiotensin I. This inactive form of angiotensin is then converted to angiotensin II, an active form of angiotensin, which can stimulate vasoconstriction and aldosterone secretion, causing the blood pressure to increase.

DISORDERS AND CONDITIONS

BENIGN PROSTATIC HYPERPLASIA

Benign prostatic hyperplasia (BPH), a common noncancerous enlargement of the prostate gland, mostly occurs in older men. BPH results in incomplete bladder emptying and urinary retention. The development of BPH is insidious, and its exact cause is not very well understood. Many factors may be implicated in the etiology of this condition.

Main Symptoms

Patients with BPH may present with symptoms of varying severity. Early signs may remain vague until urethral blockage impairs normal urination. BPH can produce generalized manifestations, such as fatigue or anorexia, as well as obstructive and irritative symptoms, including the following:

- Decreased force of the urinary stream and difficulty initiating urination
- Dribbling after voiding and a feeling of incomplete emptying
- Urinary frequency, urgency, and dysuria (difficult urination)
- Nocturia (excessive urination during the night)
- Urge incontinence
- Prostatic enlargement

Selected Nursing Tips

1. Care for patients with BPH may entail establishing the correct diagnosis, relieving symptoms, restoring urinary drainage, and preventing or treating complications. The most conservative initial treatment may include "watchful waiting" and dietary changes, such as limiting intake of urinary irritants like caffeine. Drug therapy may be prescribed, and minimally invasive procedures may be employed when deemed necessary by the healthcare practitioners.
2. When fluid restriction is implemented for bladder distension, monitor the patient for signs of dehydration. Record the patient's vital signs, intake and output, and daily weight.
3. Teach patients about Kegel exercises, and have patients practice by starting and stopping the stream several times during urination.
4. The surgical procedure known as transurethral resection of the prostate (TURP) is now performed less frequently due to the development of less invasive technologies; follow the nursing care guidelines for the specific treatment.

5. Prior to the TURP surgery, teach patients what to expect after the procedure, including some blood in the urine initially. Bladder pressure, pain, and spasm may also occur. After a TURP, a closed sterile drainage system may be used to facilitate bladder outflow and prevent clot formation that could cause obstruction and lead to disruption of the surgical site. The same amount of fluid instilled should be recovered in the drainage bag. When determining urine output, the amount of irrigation fluid instilled should be deducted from the total output.

6. Emphasize the prescribed activity restrictions after surgery, including avoidance of lifting, strenuous exercise, or long car rides; prevent constipation and straining. Sitting in a warm bath may promote muscle relaxation and reduce the risk of urinary retention.

Points to Consider

1. An elevated prostate-specific antigen (PSA) level may point to any of several pathologic conditions, including urinary retention, BPH, prostatic cancer, and infarction (necrosis due to lack of blood supply).

2. BPH is common in aging males and is not considered a predisposing factor for prostate cancer. Chronic urinary retention may, however, cause urinary tract infections and accumulation of nitrogenous wastes in the blood (azotemia), potentially leading to renal problems.

3. Alpha-adrenergic blockers, such as terazosin (Hytrin), may produce vasodilation, relax smooth muscle, and improve urine flow. Serious side effects of the medications may include dizziness, headache, and fatigue. The first dose is recommended to be given at bedtime to prevent first-dose syncope (fainting resulting from hypotension).

Precaution

Bleeding is a potential complication of prostate surgery. Before the surgery, anticoagulants should be withheld and clotting problems corrected. After the surgery, avoid rectal examination for impaction, which may precipitate bleeding (hemorrhage) and shocks. Take steps to prevent constipation.

BLADDER CANCER

Bladder cancer—that is, a malignant tumor of the bladder—may be associated with excessive exposure to environmental carcinogens and chronic inflammation or infection of the bladder mucosa. Cigarette smoking can be a major contributor to the development of bladder cancer, as cigarette smoke contains numerous cancer-causing substances. Other risk factors include chronic bladder irritation or urinary tract infection (UTI), long-term indwelling urinary catheterization, and exposure to radiation or certain chemicals, such as dyes.

Main Symptoms

- Painless hematuria (blood in urine), either microscopic or visible
- Nonspecific bladder irritability
- Dysuria (difficulty urinating) with increased frequency or urgency, possibly associated with urinary infection

Selected Nursing Tips

1. Adhere to nursing care guidelines; conduct patient teaching before and after chemotherapy, radiation therapy, and/or surgeries. Manage symptoms and monitor the patient for signs of complications.
2. Sitting in warm water or applying a warm pad may help relax the muscles and thereby decreasing the risk for urinary retention.
3. When a patient has had a stoma after bladder surgery, encourage the individual to view the new urinary stoma for better emotional adjustment, providing a mirror if needed. Teach the patient and family about stoma care per guidelines. Having a stoma should not prevent the patient from participating in most routine activities, except for heavy lifting or strenuous exercises.

Point to Consider

With the assistance of follow-up home healthcare staff or a stoma therapist, patients may better coordinate their care after surgery.

Precaution

After a cystoscopy to inspect the inside of the bladder, the patient may have pink-tinged urine and experience some burning on urination for a short period of time. Notify the practitioner promptly if the patient has chills or if bright red blood and clots appear in the urine.

BREAST CANCER

The cause of breast cancer is not clearly known. Female gender is among the risk factors for breast cancer; other implicated risk factors include family history, genetic abnormalities, hormone regulation, and excessive dietary fat intake. However, many patients have no identifiable risk factors. This section focuses on breast cancer in females.

Main Symptoms

- A hard, nonmobile, and nontender lump or mass in the breast when palpable (often at the upper outer quadrant of the breast, possibly due to this area's breast tissue type)
- A change in the size of the breast or asymmetricality
- A change in the breast skin, such as warmth, pinkish redness, or peau d'orange (orange-like thickened, dimpled skin condition) in advanced disease
- A change in the nipple with erosion, retraction, unusual discharge, or an itching or burning sensation

Selected Nursing Tips

1. Assess the patient's feelings and encourage the expression of concerns. Prepare the patient through education to increase her knowledge of the disease and treatment options.

2. Evaluate the patient's coping abilities and enlist her social support systems. Provide psychological and emotional support to alleviate the patient's fear. Educate her that having had breast surgery does not interfere with sexual function. Make the patient aware of the available community resources.

3. After axillary lymph node dissection, the patient is at risk of developing lymphedema (edema due to lymphatic obstruction), which may result from the lymph fluid not returning to the central circulation as normal, but rather accumulating in the arm. Performing the prescribed exercises, such as elevating the arm or making a fist and then releasing (muscle pumping), as recommended, may help restore the function of the arm and reduce edema.

4. Instruct the patient to protect the arm of the operated side from even minor injuries, such as a scratch. Obtain prompt treatment for any trauma to prevent complications such as cellulitis and progressive fibrosis.

5. Postoperatively, record the amounts and color of drainage; inspect the dressing carefully for signs of bleeding and report as indicated.

6. Encourage the patient to breathe deeply and use incentive spirometry, which is often prescribed, and to get out of bed as soon as possible to prevent complications as per protocol.

Points to Consider

1. Reconstructive surgery may be considered or planned before the treatment (surgery).

2. Patients of both sexes with *BRCA-1* or *BRCA-2* gene mutations may have increased risk for developing breast cancer in their lifetime.

3. Tamoxifen (Soltamox) is an antineoplastic, nonsteroidal antiestrogen agent used as chemotherapy; it may have serious side effects, including confusion or drowsiness.

Precautions

1. Instruct the patient to have routine follow-up care as recommended to detect signs of cancer recurrence.
2. The arm of the affected side should not be used for procedures, such as measuring blood pressure or giving injections.

GLOMERULONEPHRITIS, ACUTE POSTINFECTIOUS

Different terms may be used to describe glomerulonephritis based on the extent of the damage, cause, or other aspects of the disease. In acute postinfectious glomerulonephritis, there is inflammation of the glomeruli, primarily resulting from an immunologic response to endogenous or exogenous antigens, including glomerular tissue (misidentified as foreign) or bacteria, viruses, drugs, and other toxins that cause glomerular injury.

Main Symptoms

- Oliguria (diminished urine formation)
- Proteinuria with frothy urine—a sign of having proteins in urine
- Hematuria with possibly smoky, reddish urine
- Edema, initially appearing in low-pressure tissues, such as areas around the eyes
- Hypertension due to the decreased glomerular filtration rate (GFR) and other factors
- Azotemia (increased nitrogenous waste products in the blood), evidenced by elevated blood urea nitrogen or (BUN) and creatinine levels
- Nausea, vomiting, or fatigue, and other signs of acute renal failure in severe cases

Selected Nursing Tips

1. Provide vigorous supportive care to manage symptoms and treat or prevent complications; encourage rest when symptoms are present.

2. Correct fluid and electrolyte imbalances, and control blood pressure by using appropriate measures, including administering medications such as diuretics or antihypertensives, if ordered. Antibiotics, such as penicillin, erythromycin, or azithromycin (Zithromax), may be prescribed if residual streptococcal infection needs to be treated.

3. Modify dietary intake as deemed appropriate by the physician. It may be necessary to lower protein intake due to renal insufficiency and to restrict sodium or fluid intake if hypertension and edema are present.

4. Monitor lab values, fluid intake/output, and weight on a daily basis; observe for signs of acute renal failure such as oliguria, high serum creatinine levels or low creatinine clearance rate, and acidosis.

Points to Consider

1. When acute glomerulonephritis is unresponsive to treatment, it may result in chronic glomerulonephritis. This advanced stage of glomerular inflammatory disease may display symptoms such as proteinuria, hematuria, and emerging uremia (a toxic condition caused by inadequate kidney excretion of nitrogenous substances).

2. Encourage prompt treatment of a group A beta-hemolytic streptococcal infection, such as a sore throat, because streptococci may initiate an antibody formation that impairs the glomerular function.

3. In Goodpasture's syndrome, the alveolar and glomerular basement membranes are affected by autoantibodies. These autoantibodies cause symptoms reflecting immune-mediated inflammation of the lung and renal tissues, including anemia, cough, dyspnea, hemoptysis, and signs of glomerulonephritis.

Precaution

Emphasize the need for follow-up examination and routine assessment of vital signs and renal function to detect signs of recurrence of glomerulonephritis or of chronic kidney disease, including hypertension, hematuria, proteinuria, and uremic symptoms such as azotemia, nausea, vomiting, pruritus, and malaise.

PROSTATE CANCER

Prostate cancer, a common malignancy in men, usually develops slowly without exhibiting any symptoms until late in the disease. If diagnosed early, there is likely a cure. Risk factors include advanced age, excessive intake of fats, certain ethnicity, family history, and gene mutation.

Main Symptoms

Manifestations of prostate cancer may be similar to those of benign prostatic hypertrophy:

- Dysuria (difficult urination)
- Hesitancy or urgency
- After-voiding dribbling
- Urinary retention

Prostate cancer may metastasize to the lymph nodes or bones, causing other symptoms such as anemia, rectal discomfort, weight loss, or backache due to the compression of the spinal cord.

Selected Nursing Tips

1. Therapy varies widely depending on many factors, including the patient's age, health status, clinical findings, and stage of the disease. Treatment may include radiation, hormone therapy, surgery, chemotherapy, or a combination of several treatment approaches when deemed necessary by the healthcare practitioners.
2. Provide psychological support and postoperative care to allay anxiety and help maintain self-care ability. Correct fluid and electrolyte imbalances, and manage adverse effects of the therapy.

3. After surgery, patients should avoid prolonged sitting and other activities that increase abdominal pressure. While vigorous exercise should be avoided, ambulating as tolerated is advisable to prevent venous stasis and clot formation.

4. Advocate health-promoting practices and raise awareness of the high incidence of prostate cancer, especially in certain demographic groups. Educate patients about screening for prostate cancer according to guidelines.

Points to Consider

1. Some patients with early prostate cancer may not have an elevated blood level of prostate-specific antigen (PSA). An increased PSA level can indicate pathologies other than cancer. However, PSA values may be used to monitor the response to therapy, as a higher serum PSA level may be indicative of greater tumor mass.

2. While early detection may save the lives of patients with aggressive types of prostate cancer, slow-growing prostate cancer may not be the cause of death for many patients. Advise patients to discuss with their practitioners their individual needs and treatment approaches, including "watchful waiting." Many factors may need to be taken into consideration, including the patient's age, coexisting conditions, and the cancer type and stage, as well as the disadvantages of "watchful waiting," such as the risk of missing opportunities for better outcomes.

Precaution

After radiation therapy, encourage adequate hydration and monitor for signs of cystitis, such as urinary frequency, bladder spasms, or dysuria. After prostate surgery, avoid inserting a rectal tube or taking a rectal temperature.

RENAL FAILURE (ACUTE)/ACUTE KIDNEY INJURY

In acute renal failure (ARF) or acute kidney injury (AKI), there is a steady decrease of renal function over hours or days due to various causes, which may be described as pre-renal, intra-renal, or post-renal in nature. If diagnosed and treated promptly, AKI is frequently reversible. If the underlying causes are not corrected in time, it may progress to chronic kidney disease or end-stage kidney disease.

Pre-renal failure is usually associated with conditions that cause insufficient blood flow to the kidneys, thereby affecting renal perfusion (blood circulation) and reducing glomerular filtration rate (GFR). This type of AKI may result from conditions, such as dehydration, blood loss, hypotension, decreased cardiac output, sepsis, trauma, or anaphylactic shock.

Intra-renal failure is related to damage to the kidney tissue that results in impaired renal function. It may be caused by exposure to nephrotoxic agents, prolonged ischemia, or conditions that block the renal tubules or affect normal renal functioning, such as exposure to certain chemicals (e.g., the contrast agents used in medical tests) or heavy metals.

Post-renal failure, which is less common, is characterized by impeded urine output. Its causes include benign prostatic hyperplasia, prostate cancer, kidney stones, urethral edema from catheterization, and other conditions that obstruct urine outflow or cause urine to backflow into the renal pelvis, leading to renal dysfunction. Patients may have changes in urine flow or difficulty in voiding.

Symptoms vary with the degree of renal dysfunction and the underlying causes. Patients with AKI often go through initiating, oliguria, diuretic, and recovery phases. Other patients may develop chronic kidney disease, which has serious consequences.

Main Symptoms

- Imbalances in fluid and electrolytes, especially hyperkalemia (high blood potassium level) due to the kidneys' inability to excrete the body's potassium effectively or other causes, such as cellular destruction, with symptoms of muscle cramping or life-threatening cardiac irregularity

- Decreased urine output (oliguria), caused by loss of renal function, and fluid retention
- Drowsiness, headache, lethargy, and seizures
- Altered lab results (e.g., elevated blood urea nitrogen and creatinine levels)

When the disease progresses, patients may develop uremia, which affects multiple systems:

- Irritability, confusion, seizure, and neurologic symptoms
- Eventually hypertension and fluid retention, accompanied by distended neck veins or a bounding pulse
- Nausea/vomiting, diarrhea, and constipation with low serum calcium (GI absorption of calcium requires functional kidneys to activate vitamin D)
- Metabolic acidosis with Kussmaul's respirations (rapid deep breathing), which represent the body's attempt to expel excess carbon dioxide
- Dry and itching skin

Selected Nursing Tips

1. Obtain the patient's health history to help identify the underlying causes and, in turn, initiate proper treatment for the specific phase of AKI. Monitor lab values, including electrolytes, vital signs, and fluid intake/output; promptly report signs of deteriorating fluid and electrolyte status to the physician.
2. To identify causes and eliminate alternatives, on admission, find out if the patient has had exposure to nephrotoxic agents, such as aminoglycoside antibiotics like tobramycin (Tobrex), or has a history of chronic or improper use of nonsteroidal anti-inflammatory drugs, such as naproxen.
3. Bed rest may be necessary during the acute phase to reduce the body's metabolic demands. Ensure patients' safety by taking precautions against falls—they may be dizzy or confused.

4. Provide patients with small, frequent meals from the recommended diet (which commonly includes high-calorie, low-protein, low-potassium foods) and restricted fluids, if so ordered. When the patient is on fluid restriction, remove the water pitcher from the bedside.

5. Any potassium imbalance must be corrected by medication or dietary modification due to the narrow range of safety for this electrolyte. The patient may need to be on a cardiac monitor because of the risk of developing cardiac dysrhythmias or arrest. Regular insulin may be used along with glucose to move potassium into the cells, temporarily lowering the serum potassium level. Calcium replacement may also be prescribed along with other medications to treat hyperkalemia in severe cases, as calcium may help by reversing cardiac depression, protecting the heart to some degree.

6. A diet high in carbohydrate may help meet the patient's energy needs and prevent tissue breakdown; consult with the dietician for recommendations. Protein intake should be individualized to maximize the benefits and minimize the adverse effects resulting from the affected kidney's inability to excrete its end products. Intake of potassium-rich foods, such as bananas and citrus fruits, may need to be restricted.

7. Using lubricating lotion and cool water may relieve skin dryness and pruritus (itching).

8. Manage the dialysis process, and prevent complications as indicated.

Points to Consider

1. Understanding the causes of and risk factors for AKI will enable nurses to take precautions against preventable AKI; elderly patients who are confused or have limited access to drinking water are at a higher risk for this condition.

2. Blood urea nitrogen (BUN) levels reveal the kidneys' ability to excrete the end products of protein metabolism, but can be affected by other factors. Creatinine is a by-product of muscle contraction, and its blood level fluctuates less frequently. Compared with a high BUN level, a high serum creatinine level is a more reliable indicator of decreased renal function.

3. Renal creatinine clearance is another specific indicator of kidneys' function, reflecting the glomerular filtration rate (GFR). Low renal clearance of creatinine is indicative of impaired renal function, as the level of creatinine remains almost constant in the body and this substance is excreted entirely by the kidneys.

4. To prevent AKI, it is crucial to treat hypovolemic shock by promptly instituting fluid replacement as ordered.

5. For patients with renal impairment, prescribed dosages of many medications (e.g., aminoglycoside antibiotics, agents containing magnesium) are likely to be reduced because of ineffective excretion. If the patient with renal failure is on digoxin for heart failure, watch for the signs of digoxin toxicity, including GI or visual disturbances and cardiac arrhythmias. Digoxin is also excreted by the kidneys; in renal failure, the excretion of digoxin is decreased.

6. Nausea in patients with renal failure is often associated with the toxins in metabolic wastes that the kidneys are not able to eliminate.

7. In the recovery period, patients may become more lucid and less anemic, with an increase in hemoglobin level, decreased serum creatinine level, and improved GI status.

8. In patients with diabetes mellitus, routine self-monitoring and managing blood glucose, along with proper diet and exercise, are essential to prevent development of renal failure and other complications.

9. Signs of hyperkalemia include muscle weakness and ECG changes (such as tall, peaked T waves). Dialysis, hypertonic glucose and insulin infusion, and other measures may be used to treat hyperkalemia; monitor lab values closely.

10. In patients with AKI, when damaged renal tubules cannot conserve sodium, initially the excretion of sodium may increase. As urine output decreases, sodium retention is likely to occur. An increase in sodium intake can further affect fluid and electrolyte imbalances.

11. Uncontrolled dilutional hyponatremia can potentially lead to cerebral edema. Its symptoms include dizziness, weakness, and confusion. If appropriate, drinking fluids such as soft drinks or juice, instead of water, may help alleviate symptoms to some degree in certain cases.

Precaution

Monitor the patient's serum electrolyte levels closely; observe for the signs of hyperkalemia such as muscle weakness and cramping. Hyperkalemia can lead to dangerous cardiac dysrhythmia.

RENAL FAILURE (CHRONIC)/CHRONIC KIDNEY DISEASE

In chronic renal failure (CRF) or chronic kidney disease (CKD), there is a progressive, irreversible loss of renal function, affecting the kidneys' regulatory abilities. Symptoms commonly emerge when the metabolic wastes of protein, which is normally excreted in the urine, accumulate in the blood, causing uremia involving every body system. CKD can result from various conditions that destroy renal functional units (nephrons or parenchyma), leading to end-stage kidney disease.

Main Symptoms

Chronic kidney disease may produce symptoms related to physiologic changes of all body systems, varying with the stage of disease. Eventually it may cause an overwhelming array of problems:

- Electrolyte imbalances, such as hyperkalemia, which can cause dangerous or fatal dysrhythmia

- Uremia with manifestations in all body systems; waste product accumulation with high blood urea nitrogen (BUN) and serum creatinine, causing symptoms including nausea, vomiting, drowsiness, lethargy, and altered mentality
- Oliguria or anuria (when CKD worsens), and an ammonia odor to breath
- Cardiac and endocrine abnormalities, including hypertension, dysrhythmia, and increased blood glucose levels
- Anemia and bleeding tendency
- Dyspnea and Kussmaul's respirations (due to acidosis)
- GI problems, including constipation possibly due to fluid and dietary restrictions and use of phosphate-binding antacids

Selected Nursing Tips

1. Control the patient's underlying conditions; minimize symptoms or complications and slow the disease progression.
2. Patients with CKD should be advised to record daily weights and to drink the recommended amount of fluid depending on daily urine output. They should also report weight gain, increased dependent edema, and difficulty in breathing, as these are signs of cardiopulmonary involvement.
3. In early-stage chronic renal failure, patients may experience salt-wasting and polyuria (excessive urine), resulting in dehydration; carefully monitor the input/output status and replace fluid and electrolytes as ordered. When patients lose all normal renal function, oliguria or anuria (absence of urine) may occur.
4. Bathing in cool water may alleviate itching caused by uremic frost (a white layer on the skin resulting from the irritating wastes).

Points to Consider

1. Maintenance dialysis may sustain life in patients who can tolerate this therapy. Renal transplantation is another life-saving option.

2. Depending on the stage of disease, the patient with renal failure may not produce sufficient erythropoietin (a hormone necessary for red blood cell production), resulting in anemia. Epoetin alfa (Epogen) may be prescribed for patients with chronic kidney disease; its side effects may include hyperkalemia, especially in patients who are not adherent to the treatment therapy. Note that shaking the vial vigorously may denature this medication.

3. Kayexalate (polystyrene sulfonate), an anti-hyperkalemic agent, if ordered, can reduce the serum potassium level by releasing sodium ions in exchange mainly for potassium ions. One of its side effects is constipation or fecal impaction, especially in elderly patients. Kayexalate is contraindicated for patients with paralytic ileus (loss of bowel motility).

Precautions

1. Patients with CKD or end-stage kidney disease may experience metabolic acidosis. Monitor for signs of Kussmaul's respirations, as the body responds by exhaling excess carbon dioxide. If this condition is not treated, patients may develop lethargy or stupor.

2. Signs and symptoms of peritonitis—a potential complication of peritoneal dialysis—may include cloudy dialysis output, fever, abdominal pain or rigidity, nausea and vomiting, and general malaise.

URINARY INCONTINENCE

Urinary incontinence, referring to involuntary urination, may be related to many factors that affect the control of the bladder or urethral sphincter (the circular muscle around an entrance or outlet), causing leakage of urine. Predisposing factors for this condition may include urinary retention, fecal impaction, altered mobility, and some health conditions or use of certain drugs, such as diuretics.

Urinary incontinence is especially prevalent in older people. It is not a normal part of aging process, though age-related changes can contribute to the disorder.

Main Symptoms

Urinary incontinence can be described in various ways according to different etiologies or a combination of them, including:

- Stress incontinence: Involuntary urine leakage, often in small amounts, resulting from sudden increase of abdominal pressure during coughing, laughing, sneezing, or physical activities, such as heavy lifting.
- Urge incontinence: Urine leakage occurring with little warning, often large in volume, due to inability to suppress the urge of urination with or without neurologic dysfunction.
- Overflow incontinence: Urine leakage that often results from urinary retention (the bladder's inability to empty completely) when the pressure of the urine in the bladder overcomes sphincter control.
- Reflex incontinence: Urine leakage related to abnormal spinal cord functioning, with leakages occurring without warning.
- Functional incontinence: Urine leakage related to impaired awareness of the need to urinate or inability to get to the toilet in time due to mental confusion or physical limitations.

Selected Nursing Tips

1. It is important to maintain patients' privacy and self-esteem while trying to manage urinary leakage and resolve the root causes of urinary incontinence. Patients should be advised to keep a regular voiding schedule, prevent constipation, and reduce their intake of bladder irritants, such as caffeine and alcohol.

2. Exercises, especially Kegel exercises, may help reduce episodes of stress incontinence.

3. After an incontinence episode, assess the patient's bladder for signs of urinary retention. An over-distended bladder can be a cause of incontinence.

4. A voiding schedule or "bladder training" may reduce the incidence of bladder incontinence by gradually increasing voiding intervals until patients achieve acceptable patterns. Another aspect of urinary incontinence care is to manage fluid intake; if feasible, have the individual take the majority of fluids early in the day to prevent nocturia (excessive urination at night).

5. Urinary frequency can result from numerous factors—for instance, UTI, inflammation, anxiety, and incomplete bladder emptying. It is important to identify the root cause and treat the underlying condition as well.

Points to Consider

1. Pelvic floor (perineal) muscle exercises, or Kegel exercises, may help strengthen the pelvic muscles and lessen urine leakage. Simple Kegel exercises can be done dozens of times a day by tightening and relaxing the pelvic floor muscles as if trying to "start" to urinate, and then "hold" the urine stream. They can be performed repeatedly and anywhere. Some patients may achieve less urine leakage in a month or so.

2. Pain during or after voiding may be associated with bladder problems or UTI.

3. In patients with neurogenic bladder, motor-neuron problems cause them to lose the voiding urge sensation or related motor control. Provide nursing care to prevent bladder over-distension as ordered.

Precaution

Before inserting a urinary catheter or using a drainage system, verify that the patient has no latex allergy; allergic reaction to latex could be a life-threatening event. When catheterization is absolutely necessary, sterile technique must be employed to prevent urinary infection.

URINARY TRACT CALCULI (STONES)

Many factors may be involved in the incidence of urinary tract calculi or stone formation (urolithiasis). The exact causes of stone formation are not clear; predisposing conditions include stagnant urine that includes high concentrations of urinary solutes (dissolved substances in a solution), such as calcium oxalate (a salt) and calcium phosphate. Many conditions favor stone formation—for example, infection, dehydration, hypercalcemia, and immobility, among others.

Main Symptoms

Symptoms vary with the size, location, and causal factors of the calculi. The main symptom is pain, which can be excruciating at times.

Urinary tract calculi frequently demonstrate a sudden onset, with acute pain occurring on the affected side and in the flank; this pain may progress toward the groin as the stone moves downward. The pain may be accompanied by nausea, vomiting, pallor, and diaphoresis. It can be so severe that it causes vasovagal syncope, or a sympathetic response, such as clammy skin. Some patients may complain of groin or bladder pain, resulting from the referred pain of the stone.

Selected Nursing Tips

1. Assessment and pain management are priorities in nursing care. Hot baths or warm moist packs on the area may offer comfort.
2. If calcium is the main component of urinary calculi, as is the case with many stones, dairy product consumption may increase the tendency of stone formation and reduce oxalate excretion. (Oxalate is commonly present in many stones.) Vitamin D-enriched foods may also need to be limited for a while, if recommended, so as to inhibit calcium absorption from the GI tract.

3. Unless contraindicated, high fluid intake on an around-the-clock basis may increase hydrostatic pressure and aid in passing of the stones; alternatively, it may dilute the fluid enough to prevent calcium from becoming sufficiently concentrated to precipitate.

4. If the renal stone is composed of uric acid, it may be necessary to limit intake of foods high in purine, such as organ meats, chicken, and sardines. Straining all urine may assist in ascertaining if a stone is passed and determining the treatment options.

Points to Consider

1. A 24-hour urine test may be ordered for diagnostic and treatment purposes, including determining the components of the kidney stones. Before starting a 24-hour urine collection for any purpose, patients should first empty their bladder and discard that urine. All the urine within the following 24 hours (including the urine of the last voiding) should be saved and placed on ice, or refrigerated to ensure an accurate test result.

2. Adequate hydration can keep urine dilute and prevent stone formation. Dietary modification may be necessary depending on the components of the stones.

3. Allopurinol (Zyloprim) may be prescribed to reduce blood uric acid level; administer it after meals with a liberal amount of water.

4. Nonsteroidal anti-inflammatory drugs, if ordered, may decrease swelling and facilitate passing of the stone owing to their inhibitory effects on the production of prostaglandin.

Precaution

Advise patients to report symptoms of acute urinary obstruction, such as pain and inability to void.

URINARY TRACT INFECTION, LOWER

Urinary tract infections (UTIs) can be attributed to multiple etiologies. Bacterial infection due to *Escherichia coli* is a common cause, and is often seen in women. UTIs may be described in many ways, based on their location or other factors. Upper urinary tract infections may involve the kidneys or ureters; lower urinary tract infections include cystitis (bladder infection), bacterial prostatitis, and urethritis.

Any factors that compromise the mechanisms that maintain the sterility of the bladder may contribute to the development of urinary tract infection, including inability to empty the bladder completely/urinary retention, urinary flow obstruction, or medical procedures such as catheterization.

Main Symptoms

Lower UTIs may produce symptoms including cloudy urine, dysuria, frequency, cramps/bladder spasms, itching, and malaise.

Some bacteria, such as *E. coli,* are normally found in the GI tract. When bacteria in the lower urinary tract move upward into the ureters and kidneys, kidney inflammation/infection (pyelonephritis) may occur. Upper UTIs usually have systemic manifestations, such as fever, chills, and flank (side) pain.

Selected Nursing Tips

1. Educate patients on good hygiene habits, including wiping from the front to the back, which decreases the likelihood of introducing infectious organisms into the urinary tract.
2. Instruct patients to take the full course of antibiotics, even when their symptoms have subsided, to reduce the risk of inducing drug resistance.
3. Advise patients to answer the voiding urge promptly or at least every 2–3 hours. The claim that cranberry juice or vitamin C can decrease the risk for UTIs by increasing urine acidity has not been statistically confirmed.
4. Patients with frequent cystitis should, if appropriate, increase their daily fluid intake, which will help flush the bladder.

5. When a UTI is suspected, the nurse should first collect a clean-catch urine specimen for a culture-and-sensitivity test, to identify the causative organisms before initiating antibiotic therapy. A collected urine specimen should be kept at proper (low) temperature to ensure unaltered test results.

6. Older patients may not present with typical signs or symptoms of UTI. Their only manifestation may be an increase in confusion, irritability, or falls.

7. Females, in general, are prone to UTI because urethra contamination is more likely, due to the female anatomy and urethra lengths (the female urethra is approximately 3–5 cm, much shorter than the male urethra). The following measures may help prevent the recurrence of UTI in women:

   - Emptying the bladder completely every 2–3 hours
   - Cleaning from the front to the back after using the restroom and preventing constipation
   - Taking showers instead of tub baths
   - Voiding immediately after sexual intercourse
   - Judicious use of caffeinated or alcoholic beverages, as they are irritants to the urinary tract

Points to Consider

1. The cloudiness of urine is often indicative of the presence of infection.

2. Hospital-acquired (nosocomial) UTIs are often related to use of urinary catheters. When catheterization is absolutely necessary, a closed system should be maintained to prevent organisms from getting into the bladder. The drainage bag must be kept below the level of the bladder; tubing should be free of kinking to ensure free flow of urine. The catheter insertion site, surrounding (perineal) areas, collection bag, and tubing must be kept clean to prevent bacterial contamination. The catheter should be secured to the patient's leg to prevent movement-caused traction on the urethra.

Adhere to strict aseptic technique when inserting the catheter, obtaining urine specimens from the sampling port or emptying the urine collection bag.

3. Nitrofurantoin (Macrodantin) can cause urine to have a harmless brownish discoloration. Phenazopyridine (Pyridium), a urinary tract analgesic, is often prescribed for urinary pain, burning, urgency, or frequency, along with other urinary anti-infective medications. Patients should be told that this medication may turn their urine reddish-orange in color and stain clothing. Taking these two medications with food or milk may reduce GI upset.

4. Pyelonephritis, which commonly involves a bacterial infection of the kidney, may result from infection spreading from the bladder to the ureters and kidneys. Risk factors include procedures such as catheterization and conditions such as vesicoureteral (bladder-and-ureter) reflux (backward flow of urine) and urinary retention, stemming from problems including benign prostatic hyperplasia. Pyelonephritis tends to recur. Instruct patients upon discharge that follow-up urine cultures are necessary, as bacteria may be present in urine without other symptoms.

Precaution

During IV infusion of antibiotics, if infiltration or phlebitis is suspected, the nurse should first stop the infusion.

OTHER POINTERS AND CONCERNS

PERTAINING TO ACUTE URINARY RETENTION

Acute urinary retention constitutes a medical emergency that requires prompt intervention to prevent serious complications, including urinary tract infection or kidney damage. Ensure privacy and a position conducive to voiding. If appropriate, drinking a cup of coffee or tea may help maximize the urge to void as caffeine has a diuretic effect (in addition to other pharmaceutical effects such as stimulation of the central nervous system). Assisting patients to use the bathroom in a natural setting or sitting them up in a warm bathtub or shower may facilitate voiding. When other measures fail to produce results, using a straight catheter, if ordered, to aid in emptying the bladder may be indicated. However, patients with a condition such as prostatic obstruction may need to be attended to by a urologist to establish catheter access.

PERTAINING TO CANDIDIASIS

Candida (formerly *Monilia*), a kind of yeast, is commonly present in the vagina (as well as in the mouth and the GI tract). Patients who have a weakened immune system or who use corticosteroids are predisposed to yeast infection. The use of antibiotics that kill some of the good bacteria as well as the bad ones can also contribute to increased risk of developing candidiasis (yeast infection).

PERTAINING TO CERVICAL CANCER

Cervical cancer is frequently asymptomatic in its early stages. Eventually, whitish or yellowish cervical/vaginal discharge and intermittent painless vaginal bleeding may occur. As the disease progresses, patients may experience other symptoms including pelvic pain, weight loss, and anemia.

A Pap (Papanicolaou) smear test, though not 100% accurate, can be used to detect early cell changes caused by human papillomavirus (HPV) and to greatly increase cure rates. HPV infection is one of the risk factors associated with cancer of the uterine cervix and other virus-affected areas (e.g., oral cavity). Vaccination, especially when implemented at the recommended age, may reduce the incidence of cancer associated with certain HPV types.

PERTAINING TO DIALYSIS

Dialysis is a procedure used to remove toxins, metabolic wastes, and excess fluids or solutes in the blood to compensate for some of the kidneys' lost function. In hemodialysis, the patient's blood is diverted to a dialyzer—that is, an "artificial kidney" containing a synthetic semipermeable membrane that serves the functions of the renal glomeruli and tubules. The machine circulates the blood outside the body to filter out toxins as well as remove excess water. The cleansed blood is then returned to the patient.

In peritoneal dialysis, the blood is filtered at a slower rate inside the body, with the lining of the abdomen being used as a natural filter.

Common mechanisms of different dialysis treatments are based on principles such as diffusion, osmosis, and ultrafiltration.

Patients undergoing hemodialysis are at risk for bleeding due to the use of heparin to prevent clot formation and clogging of the catheter. Their coagulation status is evaluated frequently during such therapy. Hemodialysis can remove excess water or electrolytes and waste products (e.g., urea and creatinine) in the blood, but anemia may develop due to blood loss or possible red blood cell injury from the process. In addition, the dialysis process does not make up for the loss of the kidneys' endocrine function of producing erythropoietin.

Carefully take care of the dialysis access site per protocol. Patients receiving hemodialysis require routine assessment of the patency of the arteriovenous (AV) fistula that is formed via surgically connecting an artery with a vein. Check the AV fistula for the presence of bruits (swishing vascular sounds) and thrills (vibrations)—sounds produced when the arterial blood rushes into the vein. (An absence of these sounds may indicate that the fistula is not functioning as expected.) Nurses should routinely check distal pulse and capillary refill of the arm that has an AV fistula and should not take blood pressure or start an IV in that arm.

Monitor patients undergoing dialysis for adverse effects, including disequilibrium syndrome (e.g., altered level of consciousness, headache, nausea, vomiting, seizure, coma) and hypotension, a common complication of hemodialysis. The medications that are dialyzable, such as some antihypertensive agents, are usually withheld until after hemodialysis to prevent hypotension and to prevent the medication from being removed from the bloodstream during the dialysis process. The patient's daily fluid intake, urine output, and weight should be recorded.

At the end of dialysis, the patient's vital signs and hemodynamic stability are evaluated, with pre-dialysis and post-dialysis weights being compared to assess the effectiveness of fluid extraction during the process.

The major drawback of peritoneal dialysis is that it is a relatively less efficient process and puts patients at increased risk for developing peritonitis (often indicated by a cloudy return solution). Teach the patient and family to use strict aseptic technique when administering this therapy, especially when handling the catheter. Keep the dressing clean and dry, and change it as indicated to prevent infection. Using the correct technique can greatly reduce the risk of complications.

PERTAINING TO FLUID VOLUME

The balance of body fluid and electrolytes has a major impact on health and homeostasis, the state of equilibrium in the body's internal environment. Sodium plays a key role in maintaining fluid balance. In patients with fluid overload due to higher serum sodium levels, reducing sodium intake may help rid the body of the extra volume by minimizing fluid retention.

One of the indicators of fluid retention and renal status is body weight. An accurate record of weight should be obtained in patients with renal failure, using the same scale at the same time every day.

Hydrostatic pressure, or the pressure exerted by the fluid on the blood vessel walls, is the force that drives water out the vascular system at the capillary level. Conversely, oncotic or colloidal pressure (a kind of osmotic pressure exerted by plasma proteins, mainly albumin) pulls water into the circulatory system.

The difference in these two opposing forces can determine the direction of the fluid movement. Osmotic diuresis refers to increased urine output caused by a high osmotic pressure and the excretion of substances such as glucose.

PERTAINING TO GENITAL WARTS

Genital warts are caused by certain types of human papillomavirus (HPV). The diagnosis of this infection is often missed due to a lack of symptoms other than one or more warts, which are often not noticeable. HPV infection is a highly contagious sexually transmitted disease (STD).

There is no curative treatment for HPV infection, although some types are self-limiting. A preventive vaccine that protects against certain types of HPV is available.

PERTAINING TO GONORRHEA

Gonococcal infections are usually spread by direct physical contact with an infected person. They are curable with antibiotics, such as cephalosporin, when the bacteria have not become resistant to them. Indirect transmission is rare, possibly because the gonococcus readily succumbs to drying, heating, or antiseptic solutions.

Gonorrhea may cause distressing symptoms in males, but minor or no symptoms in female patients. Left untreated, complications including pelvic infection and infertility may result. Having the disease does not make the patient immune to subsequent infections with gonococci.

In caring for these patients, addressing knowledge deficits and advocating safe sex practices are nurses' significant responsibilities.

PERTAINING TO HERPES SIMPLEX VIRUS

Infection with herpes simplex virus type 2 (HSV-2) primarily affects areas below the waist level, often resulting in an eruption of vesicles in the genitals. Genital herpes is commonly transmitted through direct skin or mucous-membrane contact when an infected person is symptomatic (or through asymptomatic viral shedding). It may not produce symptoms in minor cases, especially while dormant, though fever or flu-like symptoms may occur. Viral reactivation (recurrence) may be triggered by factors such as stress, fatigue, and sunburn. Before the vesicular lesions appear, the patient may experience initial (prodromal) symptoms, such as tingling, burning, and itching at the site. Advise the patient to wear loose cotton underwear and avoid scratching to reduce the chances of secondary infection. Cool and moist compresses may ease the itching or burning.

Herpes simplex virus type 1 (HSV-1) mostly causes infections involving areas on the mouth (e.g., cold sores or fever blisters). Sun exposure or increased stress may trigger recurrent episodes.

Either HSV-1 or HSV-2 can affect the mouth and the genitals.

PERTAINING TO ILEAL CONDUITS

An ileal conduit is a surgically created channel that drain urines from the ureters, often diverting the urinary flow into a portion of the intestine that opens onto the abdominal skin surface as a stoma. An external pouch is needed to collect urine.

The urine may contain mucus when a mucus-secreting intestinal segment is used to create the conduit. Adequate fluid intake can help flush mucus out of the conduit and prevent urinary stasis and bacterial growth.

The ostomy pouch should be emptied frequently; the skin barrier is needed to protect the skin from urine irritation. If the stoma of the ileal conduit is not meticulously cared for, dermatitis, bleeding, or fungal infection may occur.

A standard (usually larger) urine collection bag may be used at night. The main purpose is to prevent urine from refluxing back into the stoma or ureters and causing adverse effects, including infection.

The obvious inconvenience involved with the ostomy pouch has led to increasing use of continence-maintaining alternatives to the ileal conduit.

PERTAINING TO INDWELLING URINARY CATHETERS

When an indwelling urinary catheter is unavoidable, strict adherence to sterile technique must be observed when inserting or changing the catheter and the urine-collecting bags. The catheter site should be routinely cleaned with soap and water to prevent contamination.

The collecting bag should be emptied before it becomes more than half full. It must be kept below the level of the bladder to prevent the urine from back flowing into the urethra, causing infection.

PERTAINING TO NEPHROTIC SYNDROME

Nephrotic syndrome may occur when the glomeruli are inflamed or damaged, causing them to become more permeable to plasma protein due to renal or systemic diseases; such a condition may lead to massive protein loss in the urine. Manifestations of nephrotic syndrome include proteinuria, decreased serum albumin (hypoalbuminemia), hyperlipidemia, dependent edema (especially on the sacrum and ankles), periorbital edema (around the eyes), and malaise. Severe hypoalbuminemia may lead to ascites, malnutrition, infection, and other serious complications.

Therapy includes correcting the underlying problems causing proteinuria, if possible. Diuretics may be prescribed to alleviate dependent edema. Sodium restriction based on the individual's status may help prevent fluid retention and reduce edema. Provide support to patients in maintaining a low- to moderate-protein diet. In patients with severe proteinuria, additional dietary protein, if so ordered or not contraindicated (when GFR and serum creatinine levels are normal), may help restore the body's plasma oncotic (colloidal) pressure, thereby reducing edema.

Nursing care interventions are often geared toward relieving edema, managing other symptoms, and treating the primary disease.

PERTAINING TO POLYCYSTIC KIDNEY DISEASE

Polycystic kidney disease (PKD), a genetic disorder, is characterized by multiple fluid-filled cysts that enlarge the kidneys, compressing renal tissue, and impeding renal perfusion, thereby affecting the kidneys' function. The clinical features and prognosis vary with the form of PKD. In the adult form of PKD, the development may be insidious, with nonspecific symptoms including hypertension and urinary tract infection or calculi. In later stages of disease, symptoms may be more obvious, including tender, distended abdomen, hematuria, proteinuria, and uremia. When a cyst ruptures, the patient may experience severe, intermittent pains.

Provide supportive care to individuals with polycystic kidney disease; implement strategies to control hypertension or pain and prevent or treat complications. Caution patients not to participate in activities that pose risks for trauma, because polycystic kidneys are highly vulnerable to injury. Genetic counseling may be indicated for young adult patients.

PERTAINING TO REJECTION OF A RENAL TRANSPLANT

Acute rejection of a transplanted kidney often occurs in the initial period after the procedure, though chronic rejection may occur over the course of several years. Careful nursing assessment may reveal signs and symptoms such as oliguria, fever, edema, and tenderness over the kidney or graft, elevated white blood cell count, deteriorating kidney function, sudden weight gain (fluid retention), and hypertension. Patients receiving certain serious immunosuppressive medications (e.g., cyclosporine) may not exhibit overt signs of rejection, other than an elevation of the serum creatinine level. Hourly measurement of urine output is crucial in assessing kidney function. Symptoms such as edema, fever, headache, and nausea may be present prior to the transplant, so they may not be pointed indicators of acute rejection.

Decreased serum creatinine levels may be an indicator that the transplanted kidney is functioning. After transplantation surgery, patients often receive immunosuppressant drugs, which may suppress bone marrow. Take precautions to reduce such patients' risk for infection by protecting them from being exposed to active infections.

PERTAINING TO SYPHILIS

Syphilis, a reportable sexually transmitted disease, is caused by a bacterium (*Treponema pallidum*). Its lesions may be highly infective; gloves and strict hand hygiene are necessary to prevent transmission of the pathogen from this source.

In some patients, the syphilis diagnosis can be missed because the initial symptoms are atypical, mimicking those of other diseases. If not treated properly with antibiotics, this disease may progress, causing irreversible damage to other organ systems.

Initially, after incubation period, the patient may develop one or more painless ulcers, known as chancres, which can occur in any skin area. If the condition is untreated, generalized infection may occur, with symptoms including lymphadenopathy (swelling lymph nodes), fever, malaise, weight loss, or sore throat; lesions may appear on the trunk or extremities. There is often a latent period, in which the infected person exhibits no overt signs or symptoms; nevertheless, early in this period the patient is still considered infectious.

If syphilis is not appropriately cured with antibiotics, late stages of the disease may seriously affect the cardiovascular, neurologic, and other systems, with dire consequences.

CHAPTER 9

Musculoskeletal Issues

The skeleton consists of 206 bones and numerous joints, which function to protect the internal organs, support body structures, enable voluntary movement, store fat and minerals, and produce blood cells via hematopoietic tissue (bone marrow).

Osteocytes, osteoblasts, and osteoclasts are three types of bone cells, each of which performs a different function. Osteocytes are mature bone cells that play a role in bone maintenance. Osteoblasts are bone-forming cells, which synthesize bone matrix. Osteoclasts are bone-destroying cells, assisting in the breakdown of bone tissue in the process of bone remodeling. The bone matrix contains collagen, minerals (e.g., calcium, phosphate), proteins, and other substances.

Bone remodeling is an ongoing process, in which bone is deposited by osteoblasts and resorbed (removed through reabsorption) by osteoclasts. This process can be influenced by a number of factors, including physical activity (particularly weight-bearing exercise); dietary intake of nutrients, especially calcium; and levels of several hormones (e.g., parathyroid hormone [PTH], calcitonin, activated vitamin D, estrogen).

Maintaining an optimal balance of these factors is key in promoting bone health and preventing osteoporosis, fracture, and other bone-related problems.

DISORDERS AND CONDITIONS

COMPARTMENT SYNDROME

There are many anatomic compartments in the extremities in the human body. A compartment in the limb is a space enveloped by a fibrous membrane, supporting the structures inside it, such as muscles, nerves, or blood vessels. Compartment syndrome occurs when elevated internal or external pressure impairs the tissue perfusion of the structures within a compartment. This condition may result from bleeding, edema, IV infiltration when the fascia cannot accommodate the increased content, an improperly fitted cast, or entrapment under a heavy object when the size of the space is reduced. The resultant ischemia may cause serious or irreversible tissue or neurovascular damage. In some cases, development of the syndrome can be delayed for a few days after the original insult or trauma.

Main Symptoms

- Deep, throbbing pain, which intensifies with passive movements
- Paresthesia (tingling sensation), suggestive of nerve involvement and neurologic compromise, often followed by numbness
- Prolonged capillary refill time with pale, dusky or cold fingers or toes, reflective of diminished tissue perfusion (blood flow)
- Pulselessness, a late sign, signifying a lack of distal tissue perfusion
- Paralysis (loss of movement), a sign of nerve damage

Any or all of these symptoms may be characteristic of impending compartment syndrome and should be promptly reported to the physician; a delay in prompt intervention may result in permanent nerve or muscle damage.

Selected Nursing Tips

1. Frequently and routinely assess the neurovascular functions of patients at risk for compartment syndrome, focusing on the "five P's": Pain, Paresthesia, Pallor, Pulselessness, and Paralysis.
2. When compartment syndrome is suspected, contact the physician immediately and remove restrictive devices to relieve the pressure on the site.

Point to Consider

Urine output should be monitored because myoglobin released from damaged muscle cells may obstruct renal tubules and increase the risk for acute kidney injury. Scanty and dark reddish brown urine can be a warning sign.

Precaution

Proper and prompt management of acute cases of neurovascular compromise or compartment syndrome is essential to prevent serious consequences.

FRACTURES

A fracture is characterized by a disruption or break in the continuity of a bone's structure. Fractures may be described based on different criteria, including their type, location, and extent, and labeled complete or incomplete, open or closed, stable or unstable, and so on. Most fractures result from trauma or accidents such as falls, but some can be pathologic, occurring secondary to a disease (e.g., osteoporosis or bone tumor) that leads to weakened bones.

Main Symptoms

- Pain
- Localized swelling, redness, warmth, discoloration, and bruising, including ecchymosis (superficial bleeding)

- Possible loss of sensation, deformity, and dysfunction of the limb
- (Possible) open wounds

The loss of pulse or function, and the presence of numbness or tingling distal to the injury site, may indicate neurologic compromise or damage.

Selected Nursing Tips

1. When assessing a new patient with a fractured extremity, focus on the area distal to the injury, including its color, pulse, and temperature. A prolonged capillary refill time (identified by pressing the nail bed with a fingertip) can indicate impaired circulation to the extremity.
2. Initially the injured limb should be stabilized. Applying a cold pack and elevating the injured limb may reduce pain and edema, and direct pressure may help stop bleeding. If blood loss is a concern, replace fluids as ordered and monitor for signs of hypovolemic shock, including increased pulse, decreased blood pressure, and cool, pale, clammy skin.
3. For immobilized patients, frequent repositioning may afford comfort and prevent pressure sores. Assisting patients in performing range-of-motion (ROM) exercises may deter muscle atrophy.
4. Adequate fluid intake can help prevent urinary stasis and renal stone formation.
5. To promote cell growth and bone repair, a diet high in protein may be recommended for patients recovering from a fracture. Vitamin D enhances the absorption and use of calcium, and promotes the healing of fractures.

Points to Consider

1. Cast care pointers:
   - Casts are used to provide temporary immobilization or stability to facilitate the healing of a fracture. To avoid

leaving a dent and causing pressure sores, no direct pressure should be applied to a wet cast (e.g., pressing with fingertips). Support the casted limb with palms or pillows.

- A cast can affect circulation and nerve function if it is applied too tightly or if edema has developed underneath the cast. For this reason, it is critical to assess and document the circulation and neurologic function of the casted body part regularly and frequently.
- In general, elevating the injured limb may reduce swelling, if feasible and appropriate. Avoid getting the cast wet, as moisture can soften it.
- The edge of the cast should be covered or padded to avoid irritation and to prevent debris from falling into the cast, causing irritation or pressure sores. Scratching or placing any foreign objects inside the cast can be harmful.
- Upon discharge, validate the patient's and family's understanding of cast care and the importance of reporting any concerns and signs of infection, such as fever, foul odor, and warmth from the cast after it is dry. An offensive odor from a cast can be an indicator of infection, requiring further assessment and intervention.

2. Hip fracture reminders:
   - Older individuals are at higher risk for hip fracture, especially women, because they often have low bone density or osteoporosis postmenopausally.
   - Fall prevention is crucial among the at-risk population, including confused and frail adults. Many falls occur when debilitated elderly people get in or out of a chair or bed. Major fall hazards include slippery or uneven surfaces, scatter rugs, and cluttered floors.
   - Compared with a forward fall, a fall to the side is said to be more likely to result in hip fracture.
   - After hip replacement surgery, routine neurovascular checks will be required. The presence of numbness warrants further evaluation to rule out neurologic compromise or damage.

- Surgical patients will have prescribed leg-position or weight-bearing restrictions to reduce complications. Pneumatic compression boots, if prescribed to prevent deep vein thrombosis (DVT), should be applied correctly according to the instructions. Exercise and ambulation of patients will be assisted or supervised soon afterward by therapists.
- When patients have been prescribed restrictions on hip flexion and internal rotation after their surgery, caution them that internal rotation or hip flexion may occur while performing daily tasks, such as putting on socks or shoes, sitting on a low (toilet) seat, or crossing the legs while seated. Encourage exercise that does not risk dislocation of a new prosthesis as directed. Remove hazardous items that will cause falls from the home environment, especially when a crutch or a walker is being used.

Precaution

At the scene of an accident, if the patient is in a safe place, rule out neck injuries and extremity fractures (or properly immobilize the suspected affected areas, a step ideally performed by trained personnel) before transferring the patient.

GOUT

Gout may be associated with an increased serum concentration of uric acid (an end product of purine metabolism) due to factors such as a genetic defect and the body's over-secretion or the kidneys' under-excretion of uric acid. Other possible causes include excessive intake of purine-rich foods such as shellfish and organ meats, conditions that disrupt the balance of secretion or excretion of uric acid (e.g., starvation), and conditions that result in rapid cell turnover and increased serum uric acid levels (e.g., leukemia and psoriasis).

Main Symptoms

- Inflammation of the great toe or other joints
- Abrupt onset of attack with excruciating pain, redness, and swelling of affected joints, often occurring at night
- Tophi (crystalline deposits), which usually develop over time in chronic gout, and involve articular or subcutaneous tissues, such as in the joints of the big toe, causing inflammatory destruction of the joints

The formation of gout tophi may result from frequent episodes of inflammation and high serum uric acid concentrations. Joint enlargement may impair joint function. With time, in the chronic stage of gout, attacks tend to become more severe and frequent, involving more joints.

Selected Nursing Tips

1. Encourage patients to make lifestyle modifications as indicated. Weight reduction may decrease the uric acid level and decrease stress on the joints.
2. Intake of purine-rich foods, especially organ meats, sweetbreads, any (red) meats, and beer, may need to be limited.
3. Adequate hydration can facilitate the excretion of uric acid by the kidneys.
4. Remind patients to avoid triggering factors, such as alcohol use, and maintain preventive habits and behaviors.

Points to Consider

1. Side effects of allopurinol (Zyloprim), an antigout medication, include drowsiness, nausea, and vomiting. Signs of hypersensitivity, such as rash, dyspnea, and hypotension, necessitate immediate action: Discontinue the administration of allopurinol and notify the healthcare practitioner.
2. Acute attacks may be precipitated by factors such as trauma, physical stress, starvation (or severe dieting), alcohol intake, and certain medications.

Precaution

In an acute episode of gout attack, pain management and avoidance of aggravating factors, such as trauma, stress, and alcohol intake, are essential. Early treatment usually yields better results.

LOW BACK PAIN

Low back pain is a very common problem, possibly due to this area's structural vulnerability and the relatively weak muscles in the lower back. Risk factors include obesity, poor posture, prolonged sitting, and improper lifting.

Main Symptoms

- Acute or chronic back pain
- Fatigue
- Possible change in gait, leg strength, or sensory perception
- Increased back muscle tone (spasm)

Selected Nursing Tips

1. Nursing care priorities may include relieving pain and fostering physical mobility. Encourage ambulation and aerobic or back exercises to maintain function, but remind the patient not to exceed the prescribed level of exercise.
2. To protect the back, it is advisable to support the back while sitting and to maintain proper posture and weight. It is also preferable to wear flat, shock-absorbing shoes and to sleep on a firm mattress in either a supine or side-lying position.
3. Discuss with patients the proper body mechanics to prevent work-related injury, such as avoiding a forward flexion position for an extended length of time, keeping good body alignment, using the large thigh muscles when lifting, and holding heavy objects close to the body to put less strain on the back.
4. Remind patients to maintain good posture by keeping the chest up, abdomen tucked in, and shoulders down and relaxed.

Points to Consider

1. Warm-up exercise may help prevent certain injuries. Walking, swimming, and yoga are examples of low-impact forms of aerobic exercise that can be beneficial for patients with low back pain.
2. Overweight may contribute to back pain by adding stress to the relatively weak back muscles.

Precaution

Unless it is required by a healing process, bed rest is often discouraged, as it can increase functional disability and awareness of pain.

MUSCULAR DYSTROPHY

There are various types of muscular dystrophy (MD), which is often characterized by progressive, symmetrical muscle weakness with increasing disability and deformity. The prognosis and symptoms vary with the type of MD depending on different (often genetic) mechanisms. Owing to better supportive care, today's patients may live to adulthood or have longer life expectancy, with specific needs to be addressed as they arise.

Main Symptoms

Muscle wasting, varying in severity, is usually progressive, even though the dystrophic muscle may become enlarged due to the deposition of connective tissue and fat. Patients' movements or the functions of involved muscles may be impaired; posture, gait, and balance may be affected as well. Patients often experience fatigue with minimal exertion and frequent falls.

Difficulty chewing or swallowing may occur in some types or cases of MD, and cardiopulmonary complications can ensue.

Selected Nursing Tips

1. Enhance patients' quality of life by addressing their emotional needs with supportive care as well as by optimizing their physical functions.

2. Participate in a multidisciplinary team effort to assist patients in obtaining needed self-help and assistive devices, such as a wheelchair or ventilation support equipment.

3. Empathize with the patient and family and anticipate their evolving needs; involve the patient and family in decision-making processes related to the inevitable course of the disease.

4. Engage the patient's participation in proper exercise, such as stretching, to delay joint contractures, muscle rigidity, and disuse atrophy.

5. Educate the patient about strategies to prevent complications resulting from immobility or incontinence, such as contractures or skin breakdown.

6. Encourage adult patients to pursue occupational training to build their confidence in becoming financially independent.

Points to Consider

1. Although no curative treatment for MD has been found to date, ongoing physical therapy with appropriate exercise and orthopedic appliances may help preserve or maximize the patient's mobility and independence.

2. Genetic counseling may be necessary for couples when a reproductive issue is a concern.

Precaution

Inform patients and caregivers of the importance of monitoring for the signs of compromised respiratory and cardiac functions, which can be potential causes of death.

OSTEOARTHRITIS

Osteoarthritis, also known as degenerative joint disease, usually occurs locally, initially as a non-inflammatory progressive joint disorder. It is especially common among elderly people, but is no longer considered a normal part of aging. Primary osteoarthritis may result from degenerative loss of cartilage related to age. Secondary osteoarthritis often results from prior injury or an inflammatory disease. While certain cases of degenerative osteoarthritis may not be preventable, avoidance of trauma or overuse of the joints and reduction of excessive body weight may decrease the risk or severity of the disease.

Main Symptoms

- Stiffness, especially in the morning upon arising
- Pain or aching, especially in weight-bearing joints (e.g., knees) upon movement (often relieved by rest), or in rainy weather in some cases
- Impaired or limited movement
- Possible bony nodules on the joints of the hand

When the cartilage covering the bone ends is lost, the pain tends to be more severe, especially with joint movement, as bones rub against each other.

Selected Nursing Tips

1. Therapy for osteoarthritis includes maintaining joint function as well as managing pain and inflammation.
2. Medication, if needed, may be combined with other methods of nonpharmaceutical pain management, such as rest, massage, and use of warm pads.
3. Encourage patients to avoid overexertion or overuse of their joints by planning and modifying their activities, and to prevent joint injuries by performing warm-up movements and gradually increasing activity intensity.
4. Aid patients in obtaining adequate nutrition and hydration, and in engaging in active/passive ROM exercises to promote optimal health and prevent contractures (e.g., fixed positions resistant to muscle mobility).
5. Be vigilant in monitoring postoperative patients for signs of compromised nerve integrity, checking their circulation status on a regular basis.

Points to Consider

1. Inactivity carries the risk of causing contractures or respiratory compromise. It is more beneficial for patients to be as active as they can tolerate. Walking with an assistive device, such as a cane or walker, as instructed by the therapist, may reduce stress on the joints.

2. After joint replacement surgery, a joint prosthesis dislocation may cause pain and movement limitation; other signs may include inflammation or drainage from the incision site. Immediate notification of the physician is indicated in such a case.

Precaution

Long-term use of aspirin, a nonsteroidal anti-inflammatory drug (NSAID), may adversely impact hearing and gastrointestinal mucosal integrity. Advise patients to report side effects such as tinnitus (ringing in the ears), a sign of ototoxicity, or black, tarry stools, a sign of GI bleeding (if it is not related to known dietary change or iron supplementation).

OSTEOMYELITIS

Osteomyelitis is a serious bone infection that is difficult to eradicate or cure with antibiotics, because the infected bone may be mostly avascular and not easily penetrated by antibiotic agents. Osteomyelitis can result from bloodborne infection, trauma contamination, or vascular compromise in some cases. Trauma patients with diabetes mellitus and immunologic disorders are especially vulnerable to osteomyelitis.

Main Symptoms

When the infection is of bloodborne origin, the onset is usually acute. Laboratory test abnormalities may include an increased white blood cell (WBC) count. Clinical symptoms may include high fever, chills, night sweats, restlessness, and malaise, which may obscure local signs. Local presentations may include swelling, redness, and warmth at the infection site; impaired movement; and relentless pain that is worsened by activity.

Selected Nursing Tips

1. Important nursing responsibilities are to take measures to prevent osteomyelitis and to educate patients regarding precautions against this condition.

2. Take steps to defend against bloodborne spread of infection from an incision, wound, or catheter placement, among other sources. Preventive measures include prompt aseptic treatment of wounds and use of prophylactic antibiotics, if prescribed, for invasive procedures (e.g., dental work) after surgery. Delaying elective orthopedic surgery while the patient has an active infection, such as a respiratory or urinary infection, may be advisable.

3. Implement repositioning, coughing, deep breathing, and exercise of uninvolved joints and muscles to ward off complications stemming from immobility.

4. Monitor for signs of worsening inflammation, such as elevated temperature or increased purulent drainage.

5. Provide a cool and quiet environment conducive to promotion of general well-being and physical strength. Encourage patients to participate in self-care activities within their physical limitations.

6. A protein-rich diet may promote healing; adequate hydration is also important.

7. Antibiotics taken on an empty stomach may enhance absorption despite possible harsh effects on the GI mucosae. Adhere to medication administration guidelines.

Points to Consider

1. Adverse effects of prolonged high-dose antibiotics (often prescribed depending on the microorganism), such as ciprofloxacin (Cipro) or cephalexin (Keflex) may include yeast infection (candidiasis) and nephrotoxicity, in addition to GI disturbances. Monitor the peak and trough levels of certain antibiotics, e.g., vancomycin (Vancocin), as required and specified to achieve therapeutic effects and minimize adverse effects.

2. Hyperbaric oxygen therapy, which is available in certain facilities, is thought to stimulate circulation and promote healing of the infected site.

3. Débridement (removal) of necrotic tissue may be performed by a physician as indicated to help clear the infection.

Precaution

Long-term antibiotic therapy may induce superinfections, including manifestations such as fever, diarrhea, pruritus, oral mucosal ulceration, or yeast infection.

OSTEOPOROSIS

In osteoporosis, new bone formation occurs more slowly than bone resorption (loss of bone mass through reabsorption). Osteoporosis reduces the patient's total bone mass and causes the bones to be brittle, porous, and abnormally susceptible to fracture, especially the vertebral, hip, and wrist bones.

Predisposing factors may include inadequate dietary calcium and vitamin D intake, estrogen deficiency (especially in menopausal women and surgically induced postmenopausal women), and physical inactivity. Secondary osteoporosis can result from a variety of conditions, including small body frame, excessive alcohol intake, and long-term steroid therapy (a major contributor), among others.

The most serious consequence of osteoporosis is fracture. Elderly people who are prone to falls are at higher risk for fractures; osteoporosis may cause pathologic fractures without any contributions from perceivable or overt stress.

Main Symptoms

Patients may be unaware that they have osteoporosis until they sustain a fracture under minor or no stress. Osteoporotic compression or fractures of vertebrae may occur over time and initially manifest as back pain and loss of height.

Patients with osteoporosis have a noticeable decrease in bone mass. Bone mineral density can be measured by a dual X-ray absorptiometry (DXA) scan.

Selected Nursing Tips

1. Promote understanding of the disease, including its prevention and treatment. Advocate ways to compensate for lowered bone density and to prevent fractures, especially in at-risk populations.
2. Ensure optimal nutritional intake, including sufficient amounts of calcium and protein. Careful positioning, proper exercise, and fall prevention (e.g., providing nighttime lights in the room and installing grab bars where necessary) are all extremely important in proactively managing osteoporosis.
3. Encourage regular, moderate exercise, such as walking, to improve coordination and curb bone loss. Weight-bearing (resistance) exercise promotes calcium deposition in the bones. Sleeping on a firm mattress and avoiding excessive bed rest are also recommended.
4. Explain to patients the negative impacts of excessive use of alcohol, carbonated soft drinks, and caffeine on bone health, and discourage smoking (help patients with smoking cessation, if necessary).
5. Teach patients about their prescribed calcium or vitamin supplementation and medication regimens; inform them of the possible side effects of such therapy.

Points to Consider

1. Several medications, such as risedronate (Actonel), may reduce bone loss (resorption) and increase bone mass in patients who are deemed likely to benefit from these medications. It is important to evaluate renal creatinine clearance level, serum chemistries, and correct electrolyte imbalance as ordered before beginning such therapy.

To minimize potentially serious side effects, such as esophageal irritation, strict observance of the (regularly updated) administration guidelines is a must. For instance, after taking risedronate (on empty stomach with a full glass of plain water), the patient should remain upright for 30 minutes (or as per updated instructions).

2. A small amount of sunlight exposure is a major source of vitamin D, which is necessary for calcium absorption and bone maturation.

Precaution

Geriatric patients are at a heightened risk of experiencing fractures as a consequence of osteoporosis. Providing teaching and enforcing fall/injury precautions are of great significance in this population.

RHEUMATOID ARTHRITIS

The origin of rheumatoid arthritis (RA), an autoimmune disease, remains unclear. In RA, the bone cartilage is damaged and the bone eroded or otherwise affected, resulting in a loss of articular surface and joint movement. The chronic, progressive inflammation of articular joints is characterized by remission and exacerbation. The onset of RA may be precipitated by stressful events, such as infection, physical exertion, or emotional depression, but no correlation has been statistically confirmed.

Main Symptoms

- Redness, pain, edema, warmth, and movement limitation, initially in the small joints of the hands, wrists, and feet
- Development of contractures, multiple subcutaneous nodules on the hands, and finger deformities
- Early-morning joint stiffness
- Systemic manifestations, including fever, fatigue, lymph node enlargement, and malaise

Symptoms often reflect the stage and severity of the disease.

Selected Nursing Tips

1. Nursing priorities may include relieving pain, explaining to patients the treatment approaches, maximizing joint function, minimizing joint deformity, and preventing complications.
2. Suggest ways to promote joint function and comfort, such as taking a warm bath in the morning to reduce morning stiffness. If there are no contraindications, swimming may be an ideal form of exercise in which patients with RA can attain maximal ROM.
3. Facilitate patients' performance of daily living activities by providing easy-to-use items, such as dressing aids, Velcro-facilitated clothing, and easy-to-open containers.
4. Advise patients to pace their daily activities and obtain adequate rest and sleep.
5. It can be beneficial for patients with RA to participate in an active exercise program within their tolerance level to preserve muscle movement and ROM. However, exercising while having painful joints is not recommended.

Points to Consider

1. In patients with RA, the antinuclear antibodies (ANA) test may be positive, indicating the presence of immune complex diseases. The erythrocyte sedimentation rate (ESR) may be increased. The C-reactive protein (CRP; an acute-phase reactant protein) assay may serve as a nonspecific test pointing to the possible presence of inflammation. Rheumatoid factor (RF) titers may be positive in many cases.
2. Heat compresses may be prescribed to enhance the circulation of affected areas and decrease pain. Safe application of such compresses should be emphasized.
3. Monitor the duration of morning stiffness, which may be indicative of the severity of the disease. In RA, nearly every system can be affected, including cardiopulmonary systems.

Precaution

Methotrexate (Rheumatrex) belongs to the class of antineo-plastic/antimetabolite, immunosuppressive medications, which have high potential for various serious toxicities. Advise patients to maintain good oral hygiene and avoid exposure to sunlight or crowds, as methotrexate lowers their immune resistance. Follow the prescription instructions carefully; handle the medication with care (or wear gloves) during its preparation or administration. Monitor lab study results and assess patients for side effects, such as bleeding and renal problems.

OTHER POINTERS AND CONCERNS

PERTAINING TO CARPAL TUNNEL SYNDROME

Carpal tunnel syndrome (CTS) commonly occurs when the median nerves passing through the carpal tunnel are compressed at the wrist. This condition causes sensory and motor changes of the hand, leading to sensations of numbness, burning, tingling, pain, or weakness. CTS is often associated with hobbies or occupations that require repetitive use of wrist movements. It may also be associated with other conditions, such as arthritis or diabetes, and with repeated exposure to extreme temperatures (thermal injuries), vibrations, or direct pressure.

To prevent carpal tunnel syndrome, it is important to identify the risk factors for nerve compression, and modify causative activities. For example, advise patients to take frequent breaks or use adaptive devices, such as special keyboard pads that relieve pressure on the median nerve. Splints or other protective applications may be prescribed to limit hyperextension and improper flexion of the wrist before invasive treatment modalities are considered.

PERTAINING TO FAT EMBOLISM

Fat embolism often results from traumatic crush injuries, especially long bone fractures, which release bone marrow fat into the bloodstream. Once in the blood, the fat may occlude small blood vessels and reduce the blood supply to major organs.

The initial sign of fat embolism may be a change in the patient's level of consciousness, such as restlessness or confusion, resulting from hypoxemia. Other manifestations may include increased pulse and respirations; wheezing; petechiae (small purplish hemorrhagic spots) on neck, chest, or arms; pallor or cyanosis; and coma.

One of the main preventive measures for fat embolism is carefully immobilizing a fractured long bone to minimize the risk of this condition. Institute other precautions, include providing adequate support for the fractured bones while repositioning patients and maintaining fluid and electrolyte balance to prevent pulmonary edema. To prevent serious complications, prompt and definitive treatment of fat embolism provided in an advanced (or intensive) care unit is vital.

PERTAINING TO HERNIATED (INTERVERTEBRAL) DISK

The intervertebral disks serve as cushions between the spinal vertebrae. Age-related degenerative changes often precede disk herniation. A herniated (slipped or ruptured) disk causes the soft cartilage portion of the disk to protrude, potentially compressing nerve roots or the spinal cord. This compression causes pain, numbness, and loss of motor function to various degrees, depending on the level of the spinal cord involved, the rate of the herniation's development, and the effect on the nearby structures. If disk herniation is untreated, permanent neurologic dysfunction may result.

In a patient with a herniated intervertebral disk, raising the straightened leg while lying supine may produce posterior leg pain. Coughing or straining may also aggravate the pain.

Bed rest, pain medication, and physiotherapy are often prescribed as conservative treatments of a herniated disk before surgery is considered.

After surgery to treat a ruptured disk, monitor the patient for signs of bleeding and swelling, which can cause compression of spinal nerves, leading to permanent neurologic damage. Remind the patient to avoid bending, twisting, or pulling motions and to maintain good body alignment (whether standing, sitting, or lying) to prevent the recurrence of disk rupture.

Postoperatively, the patient should be turned with the log-rolling technique to maintain vertebral alignment. Back strengthening exercises, as directed, are often started after symptoms have subsided. Pedal (foot) pulses should be routinely checked to monitor for signs of circulatory compromise. The nursing care plan often includes promoting mobility and reducing pain.

PERTAINING TO PHANTOM LIMB PAIN

Encourage patients who are scheduled to undergo major medical procedures such as amputation to verbalize their feelings. Provide the patient and family with emotional support, and prepare them for potential experiences to allay anxiety (without offering personal advice).

Phantom limb sensations, such as heaviness, burning, cramping, itching, or pain, are commonly felt after amputation because of the intact function of the peripheral nerves in the amputated area. Pain can be more severe when a limb is traumatically severed. Such sensations usually subside as recovery and ambulation progress.

Patients should be taught to correctly use crutches per instructions to prevent nerve damage to other body parts, such as the axillae, elbows, and arms.

PERTAINING TO STRAIN AND SPRAIN

Strain, also known as "pulled muscle or tendon" may occur due to overstretching of a muscle, frequently involving the tendon. Sprains may occur as a result of an abnormal stretching or twisting motion, often involving ligament and tendon injury with potential joint instability.

Immediately after such an injury, signs of inflammation include pain, warmth, redness, and swelling around the injury site (and possible loss of function). These signs may indicate that the body's nonspecific defensive reactions have been activated.

To reduce swelling and pain related to soft-tissue injuries, such as strains and sprains, the commonly recommended methods may be shortened to RICE: Rest, safe applications of intermittent Ice packs, Compression with a bandage, and Elevation of the body part. Application of cold packs leads to vasoconstriction, which may reduce swelling and bruising. It also alleviates pain by numbing the nerves and tissues. For a day or two, heat application is usually avoided because the vasodilation effect may cause edema or pain. In general, heat enhances blood circulation, promotes flexibility and comfort, and reduces muscle spasm and pain.

To reduce strains or sprains, it is important to perform warm-up or stretching exercises before engaging in vigorous activities. Regular strengthening, balancing, and endurance exercises are also beneficial in preventing sprains and strains. In addition, spacing the activities, wearing protective devices, avoiding extreme exertion, and being proactively aware of one's surroundings and exercise habits or risks are advisable.

Relaxation and imagery may be effective in managing pain in conjunction with medications. Proper isometric exercises may help maintain muscle strength and prevent muscle atrophy.

CHAPTER 10

Skin Issues

The largest organ in the body is the skin (integument), which comprises the epidermis, dermis, and subcutaneous tissue. Together with its appendages, such as the hair, nails, and glands, it is known as the integumentary system.

The epidermis serves as an important protective barrier. It contains keratinocytes, which produce keratin, a fibrous protein essential to the skin's protective function. The skin's melanocytes form melanin, a pigment, which primarily lends color to the skin and hair as well as protects the body from the damaging effects of ultraviolet (UV) sunlight. The external layer of the epidermis is usually renewed after several weeks. Some skin problems, such as psoriasis, occur when the cycle in which the new cells form and the dead cells slough off is disrupted or premature.

The dermis accounts for the largest portion of the skin. It provides structure, with its cells producing collagen, a strengthening, fibrous protein found in the connective tissue (e.g., the skin, bone, ligaments, cartilage) and elastin fibers that are important in skin regeneration and healing. The dermis also contains blood/lymph vessels, nerves, sweat/sebaceous glands, and hair roots.

The subcutaneous tissue, or hypodermis, consists of mainly adipose tissue (fatty cells). It protects the body through its insulation and shock absorption functions as well as attaches the skin to other tissues, such as muscle and bone.

Common skin lesion types include the following (though different terms may be used for lesions of slightly bigger size, as listed in the parentheses):

- Macules (patch), such as freckles and flat moles
- Papules (plaque), such as warts and pimples
- Nodules (tumor), which are solid, deeper masses
- Wheals, such as insect bites, which are urticarial, firm, edematous lesions
- Vesicles (bulla), such as blisters
- Pustules, such as inflamed acne lesions, which are elevated superficial lesions containing pus

Secondary skin lesions resulting from other causes include the following types:

- Fissures, such as cracks at the mouth corners
- Lacerations, which are tears of the flesh
- Excoriations, which are abrasions of the epidermis

Petechiae, ecchymosis, bruising, purpura, and hematoma are associated with hemorrhage in various degrees.

DISORDERS AND CONDITIONS

ACNE VULGARIS

Acne, which often arises from hair follicles on the face, neck, and upper trunk, is a disorder of oil-secreting sebaceous glands that are present over all of the skin surface except areas such as the palms and soles. Acne may cause lesions, including comedones (or comedos), papules, pustules, nodules, and cysts, along with an excessively oily appearance. Comedones may be called whiteheads or blackheads, depending on their characteristics.

Acne is believed to be related to occlusion of the hair follicles and androgen-stimulated production of sebum, a natural oil. It tends to occur when the endocrine glands, which influence the secretions of the sebaceous glands, are most active—typically at puberty. Genetic, hormonal, and bacterial factors may also play a role in the development of acne. Other precipitating factors include exposure to certain chemicals and irritants, emotional stress, and even seasonal changes.

Some acne-precipitated lesions may heal gradually without needing treatment. Preventing scar formation is one of the major goals of therapy.

Main Symptoms

- Oily facial appearance, with lesions arising from follicles plugged by sebum (natural oils) and keratin, on the face, neck, and upper trunk
- Closed comedones (whiteheads), covered by the epidermis
- Open comedones (blackheads), protruding and not covered by the epidermis
- Erythematous (red) papules, pustules, or cysts when comedones rupture with leakage of the follicular contents into the dermis
- Inflammatory pustules, nodules, cysts, or acne scars

Selected Nursing Tips

1. Therapy depends on the type and severity of the lesions. Management aims to combat infection and inflammation, reduce sebum production and scarring, and minimize precipitating factors.
2. Correctly used medications may have better therapeutic effects, but acne does not have a reliable cure.
3. Although diet is not believed to play a major role in the development or therapy of acne, anecdotal evidence suggests that some foods may aggravate the condition, such as deep-fried foods, cola, and chocolate or milk products.

Point to Consider

Topical antibacterial medications, such as benzoyl peroxide, clindamycin (Cleocin), and erythromycin, may be prescribed. Benzoyl peroxide gel may have an antibacterial effect, which may reduce lesions and sebum production. It can initially cause redness and scaling; some patients may have hypersensitivity or may not tolerate its use. Tetracycline will discolor developing teeth, so it is contraindicated for pregnant women and for children. Caution patients that long-term therapy with some systemic antibiotics, when discontinued, may lead to increased flare-ups and a greater likelihood of scar formation.

Precaution

Even a small amount of isotretinoin (Accutane), which is sometimes used to treat acne, is associated with severe birth defects, in addition to many other possibly serious side effects. Vitamin A can potentiate the effect of Accutane; patients should avoid prolonged sun exposure while on this medication.

ATOPIC DERMATITIS/ECZEMA

Several terms may be used to describe atopic (allergic) dermatitis, including atopic eczema or dermatitis/eczema syndrome. Atopic dermatitis is a chronic, recurrent superficial skin disorder marked by inflammation. It can afflict individuals of any age, including infants (infantile eczema). It can be allergic in nature, and is frequently associated with other allergies.

Main Symptoms

Atopic dermatitis often manifests with the following signs and symptoms:

- Pruritus (itching) and hyperirritability of the skin, with raised, red, irritated skin lesions
- Possible excoriation from scratching, with drainage and crusts
- Thickened area of the skin from chronic dermatitis
- Red, thickened, itching, and scaling lesions, which are often found on the hands, feet, arms, and legs (possibly in the adult form of eczema)

Selected Nursing Tips

1. Reassure the patient and family that eczema is not contagious; take meticulous care of the skin to prevent secondary infection.
2. Eliminate potential irritants, including use of certain detergents and physical stress.
3. Prevent excessive dryness of the skin; use tepid water and skin care items or lubricants that are recommended by dermatologists.
4. Take measures to alleviate itching and discomfort to prevent scratching and excoriation, which may lead to secondary infection.

Points to Consider

1. There is no diagnostic test for eczema. Allergic contact dermatitis can be triggered by certain plants, dyes, perfumes, chemicals, metals, or latex (e.g., latex gloves), resulting in similar lesions. Susceptibility is often genetic.
2. Latex allergy may cause a life-threatening anaphylactic response; make sure the patient is not allergic to latex before touching him or her with anything containing a latex component.

Precaution

Hot (warmer than tepid) water, skin dryness, detergent, fragrant soap, or certain lotions may aggravate the condition.

BURNS, RELATED TO

Burn injuries may be caused by different agents, such as heat, chemicals, electricity, and radiation. Improving the safety of patients' living and working environments so as to prevent burn injury is a significant nursing objective.

Elderly people are often more vulnerable to burn injury due to declines in their mobility, coordination, physical strength, and sensation or vision. Their health history and preexisting conditions or comorbidities can present greater challenges and add to the complexity of burn care. Patients with burn injuries that require special attention are immediately transferred to and treated by the experts and burn-care teams in specialized burn centers.

The Rule of Nines is often used to estimate the percentage of an adult victim's total body surface area (TBSA) that has sustained burns: The head and neck constitute 9%, the two arms 18%, the anterior and posterior trunk each constitute 18%, each leg 18%, and the perineal area 1%. A number of factors can impact the severity of burn injuries, including the burn locations, the degrees of the burns, and the affected TBSA.

The impaired capillary integrity found in severe burn injuries can cause massive shifts of fluid, sodium, and protein from the intravascular space into the interstitial spaces, seriously affecting the patient's hemodynamic stability. Treatment may proceed in multiple phases. Effective fluid resuscitation as the initial therapy is vital. Ongoing assessment and management of specific problems and prevention of complications are also critical.

Main Symptoms

Manifestations vary widely depending on the severity of the burn and multiple factors in different phases of the burn's history, including the causal agents, the burn location, the extent of the burn based on the sum total of affected areas using the Rule of Nines (or other methods of estimation), the depth or degree of the burn, the patient's general condition or vulnerabilities, and possible complications.

Outwardly, patients may present with blisters; pain; swelling; and red, white, charred, and/or peeling skin. Facial burn symptoms, including burns on the areas of head, neck, or face, a change in the patient's voice, coughing, difficulty breathing, or singed nose hairs/eyebrows, may suggest a serious airway burn.

Selected Nursing Tips

1. Assess and support the patient's airway, breathing, and circulation (ABCs) with proper measures. Be alert for signs of smoke inhalation and cardiopulmonary compromise, which can significantly increase the morbidity or mortality associated with burns.

2. Strictly observe the nursing care guidelines regarding the specific burn injury under the direction of the medical experts, who often work in specialized facilities or intensive care units. Providing prompt therapies—including proper fluid resuscitation, burn and wound care, inhalation management, and nutritional support—may improve treatment outcomes and increase survival rates. Continuous hemodynamic and ECG monitoring is usually necessary.

3. Careful management of fluid and electrolyte imbalances is of vital importance. Provide safe and timely fluid resuscitation therapy (neither under-resuscitation nor over-resuscitation) as directed by experts. Burn injuries may predispose patients to life-threatening events, including shock, renal failure, infection, hypoxia, or sepsis. Thorough assessment and timely intervention can increase patients' survival rate. In collaboration with the medical experts, the nurse's coordination of the team's actions is crucial in achieving an optimal management outcome.

4. Implementing meticulous, supportive, and comprehensive care as well as strict aseptic techniques can minimize the risks of infections and complications. Institute aspiration precautions. Carefully follow the protocols and treatment orders in caring for patients with burn injuries. Ensure adequate nutrition to further promote wound healing.

Points to Consider

1. Electrical, chemical, or other burns with different manifestations demand immediate specialized care. If a chemical has entered the patient's eyes, carefully irrigate the eyes with large amounts of saline solution or water, as appropriate.

2. Make sure the patient's tetanus immunization status is up to date, as burn wounds are often contaminated.
3. Direct application of ice to the wound is not appropriate.

Precaution

Remove restrictive clothes or items gently, possibly by wetting them with saline solution. Maintain the patient's body temperature; placement of a large, saline-soaked dressing can lower body temperature to a dangerous degree.

HERPES ZOSTER (SHINGLES)

Herpes zoster, or shingles, primarily occurs in adults. This infection is caused by the varicella-zoster virus, which also causes chickenpox. It is theorized to possibly result from reactivation of dormant varicella virus after a person has experienced chickenpox at a younger age (in some cases, without patients remembering its occurrence). Immunosuppressed individuals are more susceptible to this disease.

Main Symptoms

- Fever and malaise
- Severe pain and itching
- Blister-like lesions (vesicles) with a red base, which are often found on one side of the face, trunk, or thorax

Selected Nursing Tips

1. Provide supportive treatment to relieve itching and pain. Keep the patient comfortable with diversionary activities as preferred, while ensuring adequate rest periods during the acute phase.
2. Cold compresses may have a soothing effect on areas populated with vesicles, decreasing the patient's urge to scratch and, in turn, preventing infection.
3. Offer the patient a soft diet and soft toothbrush if oral lesions are present.

4. Administer analgesics exactly on time per the dosage schedule to prevent the pain from becoming too severe. Patients may experience intense pain, especially associated with the eruption of the lesions and formation of scabs.

Points to Consider

1. The disease is benign in most cases, but serious complications can occur. A vaccine is available to decrease the risk of developing shingles.
2. If patients have been prescribed antiviral agents, such as acyclovir (Zovirax), to reduce pain or possibly halt the progression of the infection (when the therapy was initiated shortly after the rash eruption), watch for signs of these agents' side effects or toxicity, such as nausea or malaise. Adhere to the prescribed infusion rate; rapid administration can cause renal tubular damage. Ensure adequate hydration during and after infusion. Patients with a compromised renal system (and therefore slower excretion of the drug) are more vulnerable to toxicity.
3. If patients continue to take narcotic analgesics after the period when they suffer herpetic neuralgia (intense pain along the course of the nerve), caution them about the increased risk of addiction.

Precaution

When an eye is affected by herpes zoster, it is an ophthalmic emergency. The patient should be immediately referred to an ophthalmologist to prevent serious complications, including ulceration or even blindness.

LYME DISEASE

Lyme disease is a tick-carried multisystem disorder, which was first identified in Lyme, Connecticut. It is caused by the bite of an infected tick that feeds on both animals and humans, but is not transmitted from person to person. If not treated promptly, this infection can progress, affecting other systems with cardiac, neurologic, and other abnormalities.

Main Symptoms

The symptoms of Lyme disease may present in several stages. Initially, within days or weeks, a "bull's eye" red rash may develop slowly, primarily at the site of the bite; it may be accompanied by flu-like symptoms, including fever, chills, malaise, swollen lymph nodes, and joint and muscle aches. The rash eventually subsides even without treatment.

If antibiotic therapy is not initiated in time, over the course of weeks or months the patient may display systemic symptoms. These symptoms mimic those associated with other diseases and may include arthritis-type pain and swelling in the large joints, poor motor coordination, and memory loss. Serious neurologic deficits, including confusion, may develop long after the initial bite. Chronic or recurrent sequelae may also occur, even years later, potentially resulting in permanent disability.

Selected Nursing Tips

1. Elicit the patient's travel history, including outdoor activities in potentially tick-inhabited areas. Teach the patient about the symptoms and the possible course of Lyme disease.
2. Carefully assess the lesion to rule out other causes of rashes. Follow the treatment protocol, and monitor lab results and treatment therapy. Emphasize the need for the patient to commit to follow-up appointments.
3. Initiate antibiotic therapy when ordered. Instruct the patient how to comply with this treatment regimen, including maintaining a consistent dosing schedule, finishing the full prescribed course, and reporting side effects and responses.
4. While engaging in outdoor activities, be aware of the risks and avoid being exposed to ticks to prevent Lyme disease.

Point to Consider

Culture or other lab methods are not frequently used to identify Lyme disease prior to beginning treatment, as it takes too much time to get results from the culture of the disease-causing organism or detect antibodies with tests such as enzyme-linked immunosorbent assay (ELISA) or Western blot.

Precaution

Advise the patient with a suspected tick bite to seek prompt treatment; early treatment is essential to prevent serious complications.

PRESSURE ULCERS

Pressure ulcers, or bedsores, often occur over bony prominences as a result of unrelieved pressure (for approximately 1–2 hours), which may impede normal blood flow to the area, causing tissue ischemia or swelling. The inflammatory reaction may lead to ulceration or ischemic cell necrosis, which predisposes the patient to bacterial infection. The severity of tissue damage may be governed by the intensity and duration of such pressure and the patient's susceptibility to this condition. Individuals who have compromised health status and are immobile can be at high risk for developing pressure ulcers, especially when they are malnourished, confused, or incontinent.

Main Symptoms

Pressure ulcers most frequently develop over bony areas where prolonged pressure is likely to be sustained. A specific estimated "stage" may be used to describe the degree of pressure-related tissue damage (aside from other symptoms), depending on the skin and tissue affected. However, pressure ulcers may not be accurately assessed with staging criteria because the true depth of the lesion is sometimes difficult to determine. The intensity and duration of the pressure exerted on the skin and the patient's condition can also affect the severity of the lesion.

Selected Nursing Tips

1. Identify risk factors in debilitated patients who are predisposed to pressure ulcers; take preventive measures, such as posting a turning schedule to ensure frequent position changes, providing meticulous skin care, and implementing pressure relief alternatives, such as use of paddings.

2. Establishing a routine to assess the skin for signs of compromised integrity and promptly addressing skin problems are essential in preventing the development of pressure ulcers.

3. Handle patients gently. Avoid pulling patients while turning or sitting them up, and use a draw sheet as an aid, if necessary, to prevent friction.

4. Administer passive range-of-motion exercise if patients are unable to exercise on their own.

5. Perform wound care or dressing changes as instructed by the physician or wound care expert.

6. A high-protein diet with vitamins (especially vitamin C), minerals, and adequate fluid may promote healing of the damaged skin tissue.

Point to Consider

Raising the head of bed to more than 60 degrees may create a shearing force, posing a risk for developing pressure sores.

Precautions

1. Immobile patients need to be repositioned at proper intervals to stave off prolonged pressure on skin tissue, especially over bony prominences. Performing frequent skin assessments can help prevent deep ulcers from going undetected; skin penetration of a pressure ulcer may become visible at a later stage of development.

2. Avoid using skin care agents that are harmful to the skin of patients predisposed to pressure ulcers, such as harsh alkali soaps and detergents.

PSORIASIS

Psoriasis, a recurrent noninfectious skin disorder, is characterized by raised, red, round lesions covered with silvery scales (resulting from excessive, rapid turnover of epidermal cells). This condition has a hereditary tendency, though its exact cause remains unknown. Many factors seem to be associated with exacerbation of psoriasis, including stress, skin injuries, and sunlight (UV damage). It may cause serious complications, potentially involving a large body area and one or more joints such as arthritis.

Main Symptoms

- Profuse red, raised patches covered with silvery scales, often occurring bilaterally on the scalp, chest, elbows, knees, lower back, or nails
- Pruritus (itching)
- Occasional pain from dry, encrusted lesions
- Bleeding spots seen when the crusts of lesions are removed

Selected Nursing Tips

1. Therapy depends on the size of the affected area and the severity of the lesions. Assess patients' coping mechanisms, and reassure them that psoriasis is not a result of poor hygiene, and that it is not contagious or cancerous.
2. Suggest alternative stress-reduction methods, including relaxation, exercise, good nutrition, and rest to boost immune status.
3. Help patients to be aware of provoking factors, including skin irritation or injuries and emotional stress.
4. Educate patients about proper application and side effects of prescribed topical medications, such as corticosteroid creams or ointments; caution patients not to discontinue any steroid medications abruptly.
5. Recommend ways to increase skin integrity: Keep the skin moist by using a proper cleansing agent or moisturizer, as dry skin aggravates a psoriatic condition; use lukewarm (instead of hot) water; and pat the skin dry.

Points to Consider

1. Even though exposure to sunlight may worsen the condition, a controlled amount of ultraviolet-B (UVB) light is often the therapy used to decrease the epidermal-cell growth rate so as to treat psoriasis. Teach patients about treatment regimens according to the specific instructions given by the therapist, such as wearing goggles when exposed to ultraviolet (UV) light during the therapy session.

2. Treatment approaches are basically symptomatic and palliative—that is, they alleviate the symptoms of psoriasis but do not cure it. The use of systemic corticosteroids is limited due to the risk of serious flare-ups upon its discontinuation. It is important to minimize the side effects of the treatments, boost the patient's general health, and avoid precipitating factors.

Precaution

Caution patients who receive UV light treatment to avoid sun exposure, and to wear eyeglasses or shields to protect the eyes as instructed by the therapist.

SCABIES

Scabies is a highly contagious skin disease caused by itch mites. It is transmitted through skin contact. Individuals with limited physical ability to maintain adequate hygiene and those who are living in a crowded environment are more susceptible to outbreaks of scabies.

Main Symptoms

- Small, raised, red, threadlike lesions (burrow-tunnels made in the skin by mites), commonly seen on the wrists or between the fingers, but possibly not visible
- Intense itching, especially at night
- Excoriations due to scratching or secondary bacterial infection, with vesicles or crusts

Selected Nursing Tips

1. Thoroughly disinfect any contaminated items and the patient's room, including washing clothing and bedding in hot water and then drying these items with a hot dry cycle.
2. To contain the spread of the disease, take strict infection-control measures by practicing meticulous hand washing and wearing gloves. Close contacts of the patient should be treated simultaneously.
3. Strictly follow the instructions when using a scabicide agent; avoid applying the medication to the face, any mucous membranes, and any excoriated (raw) or inflamed areas. The agent should be washed off thoroughly according to the instructions, within the time frame recommended by the manufacturer.

Point to Consider

Geriatric patients may not exhibit the same inflammatory reaction as is typically seen in younger people.

Precaution

Lindane (Kwell) has various contraindications; strictly adhere to the application instructions if it is prescribed.

SKIN CANCER, RELATED TO

Various terms may be used to describe skin cancers involving different skin-cell types, which may demonstrate different characteristics. Non-melanoma skin cancers frequently develop in sun-exposed areas of the skin. The exact cause of melanoma is unclear, but over-exposure to UV radiation, including artificial tanning booth treatments, can be a serious risk factor. Melanoma has the potential to metastasize to any organ through the blood and lymphatic routes, including to the lungs and the brain.

Main Symptoms

Basal cell carcinoma commonly develops on sun-exposed areas, especially on the face. Initially, it may take the form of a small, smooth, translucent, pigmented papule or nodule, but it eventually becomes an ulcerative lesion.

Squamous cell carcinoma can be invasive. It may appear as a rough, scaly, and possibly inflamed or bleeding tumor. Exposed upper extremities and facial areas are common sites for such carcinomas.

Different types of malignant melanoma differ greatly in their clinical presentations and other aspects. In general, the ABCD mnemonic may be used as a reminder when assessing a suspected melanoma:

- Asymmetric lesion with uneven elevations
- Border irregularity
- Color with various shades of red, white, and blue within a lesion
- Diameter greater than 6 mm (not a significant sign, as early-stage melanomas can be smaller)

Selected Nursing Tips

1. Advocate skin cancer prevention, regular sunscreen application, and routine skin examination. Closely watch for changes in the size and color of any moles, including using the ABCD mnemonic as a reminder.
2. Informing patients, when applicable, of the risk and predisposing factors for skin cancer can be one of the nurse's functions.
3. Teach self-care skills after treatment (e.g., excision or radiation) and prevention of cancer recurrence.
4. Advocate for safe sun exposure and routine use of sunscreen products recommended by dermatologists, which often include those labeled as "broad-spectrum" agents.

Points to Consider

1. Sunscreens are rated according to the sun protection factor (SPF), which measures their effectiveness in filtering or blocking UVB radiation.
2. Patients can be taught to use the ABCD mnemonic to monitor their skin lesions. Advise them to seek further evaluation if a lesion such as a mole becomes **a**symmetrical with an irregular **b**order or **b**leeding, darkened or changing in **c**olor, and increased in **d**iameter.

Precaution

Sun exposure can cause degenerative changes in the skin. UVB radiation is believed to have carcinogenic effects, and ultraviolet-A (UVA) radiation adds to that effect. Many skin cancers are thought to be directly or indirectly induced by prolonged sun exposure, damage from which is cumulative in nature.

Selected Bibliography

American Stroke Association. *Together to End Stroke*. Dallas, TX: American Stroke Association; 2016.

Beers MH, Berkow R, eds. *The Merck Manual*. 17th ed. Whitehouse Station, NJ: Merck Research Laboratories; 1999.

Billings DM. *Lippincott's Content Review for NCLEX-RN*. Philadelphia, PA: Wolters Kluwer Health/Lippincott Williams & Wilkins; 2009.

Billings DM. *Lippincott's Q & A Review for NCLEX-RN*. 9th ed. Ambler, PA: Wolters Kluwer/Lippincott Williams & Wilkins; 2008.

Boyd D, Hinds MM, Hyland JR, Saccoman EA, eds. *Comprehensive Review for the NCLEX-RN Examination*. 2nd ed. St. Louis, MO: Mosby Elsevier; 2008.

Colgrove KC, Callicoatt J. *Med-Surg Success*. Philadelphia, PA: F. A. Davis Company; 2007.

DiGiulio M, Jackson D, Keogh J. *Medical-Surgical Nursing Demystified*. New York NY: McGraw-Hill; 2007.

Hargrove-Huttel RA. *Medical-Surgical Nursing*. 4th ed. Ambler, PA: Lippincott Williams & Wilkins; 2005.

Hennessey IAM, Japp AG. *Arterial Blood Gases Made Easy*. Edinburgh, UK: Churchill Livingstone Elsevier; 2007.

Hoefler PA. *The Complete Q & A for the NCLEX-RN Exam*. 5th ed. Burtonsville, MD: Medical Education Development Services; 2004.

Hogan MA, Davenport J, Estridge S, Zygmont D. *Medical-Surgical Nursing: Reviews and Rationales*. Upper Saddle River, NJ: Pearson Education, Inc.; 2008.

Hood GHH, Dincher JR. *Total Patient Care: Foundations and Practice of Adult Health Practice*. 8th ed. St. Louis, MO: Mosby-Year Book; 1992.

Ignatavicius DD, Workman ML, eds. *Medical-Surgical Nursing: Patient-Centered Collaborative Care*. 7th ed. St. Louis, MO: Elsevier Saunders; 2013.

Irwin BJ, Burckhardt JA. *NCLEX-RN Exam*. New York, NY: Kaplan Publishing; 2006.

Kizior RJ, Hodgson BB, Hodgson KJ, Witmer JB. *Nursing Drug Handbook 2015*. St Louis, MO: Elsevier Saunders; 2015.

Laskowski-Jones L, Gasda KA, Carey KW, et al. *Nursing 2016*. Philadelphia, PA: Wolters Kluwer; 2016.

LeMone P, Burke KM. *Medical-Surgical Nursing: Critical Thinking in Client Care*. Menlo Park, CA: Addison-Wesley Nursing; 1996.

Lewis SL, Dirksen SR, Heitkemper MM, Bucher L. *Medical-Surgical Nursing: Assessment and Management of Clinical Problems.* 9th ed. St. Louis, MO: Mosby Elsevier; 2014.

Lippincott Williams & Wilkins. *Handbook of Diseases.* 3rd ed. Philadelphia, PA: Lippincott Williams & Wilkins; 2004.

Lippincott Williams & Wilkins. *NCLEX-RN: Review Made Incredibly Easy.* 5th ed. Ambler, PA: Wolters Kluwer/Lippincott Williams & Wilkins; 2011.

Lippincott Williams & Wilkins. *Portable RN: The All-in-One Nursing Reference.* 4th ed. Ambler, PA: Wolters Kluwer/Lippincott Williams & Wilkins; 2011.

Lippincott Williams & Wilkins. *Springhouse Review for NCLEX-RN.* 6th ed. Philadelphia, PA: Lippincott Williams & Wilkins.

Lippincott Williams & Wilkins. *Straight A's in Medical-Surgical Nursing.* 2nd ed. Ambler, PA: Wolters Kluwer/Lippincott Williams & Wilkins; 2008.

Lisko SA, ed. *NCLEX-RN: Questions & Answers Made Incredibly Easy.* 7th ed. Philadelphia, PA: Wolters Kluwer; 2017.

Oglesby RC, ed. *NCLEX-RN Review.* 6th ed. Clifton Park, NY: Delmar Cengage Learning; 2010.

Ohman KA. *Davis's Q & A for the NCLEX-RN Examination.* Philadelphia, PA: F. A. Davis Company; 2010.

Pagana KD, Pagana TJ. *Mosby's Manual of Diagnostic and Laboratory Tests.* 5th ed. St. Louis, MO: Mosby Elsevier; 2014.

Saxton DF, Nugent PM, Pelikan PK, eds. *Mosby's Comprehensive Review of Nursing for the NCLEX-RN Examination.* 19th ed. St. Louis, MO: Mosby Elsevier; 2009.

Saxton DF, Pelikan PK, Nugent PM. *Mosby's Review Questions for NCLEX-RN.* 4th ed. St. Louis, MO: Mosby Elsevier; 2001.

Silvestri LA. *Q&A Review for the NCLEX-RN Examination.* 4th ed. St. Louis, MO: Saunders Elsevier; 2009.

Silvestri LA. *Comprehensive Review for the NCLEX-PN Examination.* 4th ed. St. Louis, MO: Saunders Elsevier; 2010.

Skidmore-Roth L. *Mosby's Nursing Drug Reference.* St. Louis, MO: A Harcourt Health Sciences Company; 2002.

Smeltzer SC, Bare BG, Hinkle JL, Cheever KH. *Textbook of Medical-Surgical Nursing.* 12th ed. Philadelphia, PA: Wolters Kluwer/Lippincott Williams & Wilkins; 2010.

Smith SF. *Review Questions for the NCLEX-RN.* Stamford, CT: Appleton & Lange; 1997.

Swearingen PL. *Manual of Medical-Surgical Nursing Care.* 6th ed. St. Louis, MO: Mosby Elsevier; 2007.

Van De Graaff KM, Fox SI. *Concepts of Human Anatomy and Physiology.* 4th ed. Boston, MA: William C. Brown Publishers; 1995.

Venes D. *Taber's Cyclopedic Medical Dictionary.* 21st ed. Philadelphia, PA: F. A. Davis Company; 2009.

Zerwekh J, Claborn JC, eds. *Illustrated Study Guide for the NCLEX-RN Exam.* St. Louis, MO: Mosby Elsevier; 2010.

Index